Forget the Cures

Find the Cause

Book One

RAYNA M GANGI

Outskirts Press, Inc.
Denver, Colorado

Forget The Cures, Find The Cause
Book One
All Rights Reserved
Copyright © 2006 Rayna M. Gangi

Outskirts Press
http://www.outskirtspress.com

ISBN-10: 1-59800-698-3
ISBN-13: 978-1-59800-698-8

Outskirts Press and the "OP" logo are trademarks belonging to Outskirts Press, Inc.

Printed in the United States of America

ACKNOWLEDGEMENTS

My mother, Ruby Krautsack, who always expects another book. Without her, I wouldn't be.

Julia Meyerowitz, a gift from God. Without her, my heart and soul would be much weaker

Without the unconditional love of those around me, there would be too few commas, not enough spirit, an entirely different voice, and most importantly, possibly no book at all.

Laurie Azzarella played one of her favorite roles and made sure she challenged my intention, which ensured my commitment to body, mind, and spirit. Without her, the book would remain an idea.

Elsa Claverie spent countless hours making sure my grammar was as close to correct as possible. Without her, there would be no words.

Renee Garrett stayed up past her bed time many times to listen to the next ten pages. Without her, there would be no voice.

Phoebe Jackson rushed to each appointment to peruse the next chapter and identify with different processes. Without her, there would be no flow.

I am always grateful to those in my life who give freely from their hearts, share their minds, and bare their souls.

All of you are forever loved.

INTRODUCTION

The purpose of this book is not to diagnose, provide home remedies or magical cures, prescribe medication, or to frighten you. As a Holistic Health professional, I've seen too many suffer from false hopes and phony claims. Maybe I'm just like you. Maybe I've had enough of the medical profession's condescension, the pharmaceutical companies peddling any drug they can come up with, and the natural healing gurus who use allopathic ideology in their multi-level sales plans. Maybe I'm tired of seeing people hoping for the one pill, one drink, or the one answer that will cure all their pain or save a loved one from death. We don't need books and pills claiming miracle cures. We don't need the newest "discovery" promoted on infomercials. We don't need to feel helpless or afraid or defeated. We need to find the causes. When we learn enough about ourselves to get to the root of any health problem, the cures will be unnecessary.

I grew up in the fifties when lake water was still almost safe for swimming and chlorine in the drinking water was supposedly taken care of by the Culligan man. Childhood gave us vaccinations because frightened parents didn't want their children to get polio or smallpox. We took antibiotics at the first sign of a bad cold and aspirin for a fever. Drugs got us back to school and doctors who asked questions, knew your history and made house calls became legends. Whenever we didn't feel well, we knew someone had a cure or a remedy. As children, we believed in Mom and doctors, and even though we didn't always want to take our medicine, we did. We never thought about the consequences or long-term effects. It wasn't our job.

As we got older, we discovered health food stores and fitness magazines with articles proclaiming miracle foods and supplements that would keep us young and strong. Somehow, we believed we'd never age, and if we went to the gym or health spa, took our vitamins, and swallowed our medicine when we were sick, nothing could stop us.

When we started having kids of our own, our presumed wisdom and years of experience gave us all the answers. Antibiotics, Asthma medication, children's aspirin for a fever, cough medicine for allergies, inhalers when necessary, even antidepressants if the doctors said our kids needed them, all became routine. When friends or family members recommended a new herb or a better vitamin, we hardly questioned their opinions. When magazines or health professionals clumped our children into groups and labeled them asthmatics or ADHD, we allowed it. After all, they knew best, and we were far too busy to delve into the complicated world of balanced health. It still wasn't our job.

Nowhere, except in paraphrased research articles from pharmaceutical companies or media advertisements from drug stores, did we ever hear the word "cause," when it came to illness. Even then the definition of the word was distorted. We caught colds from someone's sneeze and were destined for catastrophic illness because our parents or grandparents handed down the genes. When we went to the miracle workers for help, they gave us the cure, not the cause. The symptoms were far more important than the reason. When symptoms reappeared, we took stronger drugs or found a different doctor. No one heard the little voice saying, "Find the cause."

Bookstores and the Internet are packed with health and fitness books, each one touting a different approach to symptoms and pulling us in for the sale by promising cures that no one else will tell you. Health food stores are now on every corner pushing organic food, supplements, and fruit smoothies so we can feel better, or believe we do. The alternative health professions are booming and the country's masses of massage therapists, nutritional gurus, spiritual leaders and specialists promise us they have the way to happiness and heaven. Still they treat the symptoms. From depression to obesity to something coined bi-polar, there is a pill, a drink, or an herb that will cure it. With the millennium, health food owners evolved into pseudo-doctors, purchasing computer programs that can purportedly read the eyes and then tell you which vitamins and other supplements you need to buy from them to cure the problem.

The medical profession also evolved. Once they were only a handful of men who continuously passed their theories back and forth and never got creative in finding causes. Hippocrates told them to do no harm, and that the reason for all disease could be found in the spine and in our food. Though he was observant with patients and asked many questions to get to a cure he, too, soon forgot there must be a reason. After the plague killed millions of people in Europe, doctors had to recreate themselves. There were no books or theories on such a disease, no references to fall back on, no one to ask. They had to research what might have caused this terrible tragedy. With that research came prevention, and with the idea of preventative medicine came inoculations and drugs. Research became the key, not for the true cause of illness, but rather for the synthetic, manmade, laboratory solution to change or alleviate symptoms. If all else failed, they resorted to surgery, as it was the scalpel, amputations and brain surgery that began their evolution from the Middle Ages. What doctor today doesn't follow the path of medicate or operate?

So what is the answer? Another book of false hopes,

touted cures and folk remedies? Another discourse on one person's path to wellness that now everyone should follow? Another list of common illnesses and the cleanses, supplements and herbs everyone needs to try? How about antagonism or fear as motivation for another sale?

Doctors are not out to harm you or to kill you, but they come from fear more than love in their analysis and treatment protocols. Fear they will be sued. Fear there haven't been enough studies or research to justify their treatments. Fear as a culture that has too long been trained to rely on others for their knowledge, rather than educating and trusting the patient.

I intend to teach you about yourself and the world you are a part of. I hope to help you understand your body, mind and spirit in a way that no one specialist can ever approach. My passion is your health, and with that passion comes the commitment to help you overcome everything you've been taught about your body, your mind, your spirit, your health, and the health of your family. That commitment comes from love, not fear, and the love comes from more than forty years of earth medicine education, alternative and complementary health practice, and a God that has helped me and others to help so many.

CHAPTER I

U nderstanding holistic health means understanding your roots and your connection to Earth and Heaven. The Earth, we've been taught, is one of nine or more planets in a solar system. It has a history, a geology, a topography and many electro-magnetic forces that create and allow life. It has layers of composition consisting mainly of water and minerals and its core is a mystery to all but the most creative science fiction writers. We know it is somehow connected to God, or whomever we believe created it, and it changes every day. It has within its power the ability to cleanse its rivers and streams, move its magnetic plates and nourish those who live within and on it.

The Earth also has the power to self-destruct and to struggle for survival. It reacts to change, poisons, and man-made obstacles. It dies without water and gasps when it cannot breathe.

It has rainbows and stars and warming sun that smiles at us in the morning. It sings, helps birds to soar, cushions our fall, provides our food and heals our wounds. Look in the mirror. Aren't we all a part of this wonder? Don't we also have a history, a genealogy that gives us our birthmark and clues to our beginning? Aren't we all topographic, in different shapes, sizes and colors?

The Earth is 75-80% water. So are we. The Earth's minerals are the same elements that compose the tissues, blood and bones of our bodies. Each of those elements has either a positive or a negative charge and reacts to the magnetic poles and electro-magnetic forces within and around us. Our physical selves are very much like the Earth we walk on.

We separate ourselves from the Earth with our minds, of which we consciously use only 8 to 12 %. The mind allows us to create, and provides the stimulus to a network of wires we call nerves to give us movement and the ability to change shape. We can change our minds as quickly as the magnetic forces within us can change direction. We can alter our minds with drugs and close our minds with prejudice, judgment and bigotry. We can open our minds to new ideas, new places, new experiences, and seal our minds when our egos are challenged or afraid. The mind and the body are a team, and what we think or believe is reflected in our body language, our walk, our stance and our vision. We see and hear what we want to and physically react to loud noises, violent attacks or sad stories. As children, we cried or peed in our pants when we saw or heard something frightening. Out of trust, we allowed our minds to be controlled by radio and television, advertising, and the misguided wisdom of others. Because we gave up the power to reason for ourselves and have stayed too afraid of the world, or Hell, or the wrath of God, we have also lost the power to unconditionally love ourselves and others. We're no longer in charge of our health or happiness. How often do we chide the person who has "a mind of his own?" Are we so afraid? Have we been taught so well to fear instead of love that we no longer resemble the precious and unique individuals we were intended to be? There are only two emotions that truly exist in our lives, fear and love. Emotions are energy in motion. All feelings, thoughts and actions can be reduced to one question. Are we coming from fear or from love? If we are coming from fear, we have a responsibility to face it, overcome it, or change ourselves so we come only from love.

Does the Earth have a soul or a spirit, as we believe we do? Is there anyone who doesn't believe there is a part of us that's untouchable, unknown, unrealized? We have free will, a gift, and the power to choose, but what part of us knows the outcome and the reason? Our spirit is a complicated energy, an appendage of a God that knows all. A whisper, a breeze, a fall day, an eagle's cry, a baby's smile – with each we feel something in our souls. We search for soul mates through dating services or parties and long for the forever relationship that we believe completes us. We attach the heart to the soul in songs and greeting cards, knowing somehow that love is connected to soul and that soul is a good thing. For some there are spirit guides, to others angels, and still others unseen teachers who have the key to our soul and our purpose and help us on our paths. Indeed the Earth has a soul. It, too, is a unique creation, entrusted with our well-being, unconditionally providing food, water and life, and somewhere deep inside knowing its purpose.

Holistic health, or the wholistic approach to health, considers all of these things when dealing with imbalance. There is no drug or cure for a broken heart, but there are questions to be asked, patterns to be discovered, physical reactions, mindful changes, and spiritual comforts. To approach the body holistically is to encompass and respect the whole being. Our creation began long before our conception and birth. Healthy, balanced parents, both mother and father, are essential to a baby's well-being. If one parent abuses alcohol or drugs, our children will be affected and thus the grandchildren. If one parent takes over-the-counter medications on a regular basis, our livers and interstitial tissues hold the memory. If we are conceived in anger, with guilt, without love, we will live those lessons, and possibly inflict others with the projection of those negative feelings and thoughts. No one of us is alone. No one's life is untouched by others. Each of us is part of a continuous circle, each life cycle learning and building on the one before.

When approaching someone holistically for the first time my initial questions, other than birth date, name, and present residence, are birthplace, parent's birthplace, residence as a child, and all the moves in between. We need to know that the geology, water tables, plant life, homegrown vegetables, air and environment differ in all parts of the country, all parts of the world. We may have been healthy until we moved to Florida or California. We felt fine until we changed our drinking water. Nothing bothered us until that one ski trip when we fell or the car accident when we didn't think we were hurt. The timelines become vital in the slow journey back to the cause.

My next questions center around the present, what the mind perceives as the pain or problem. Our minds hold information and perceptions, but sometimes also hold back important facts that we have chosen to forget. We know we hurt, but there's no reason, or so we believe. Nothing has happened to cause any problems. We're just sick or know we're not well. When we visit doctors, we're very ready to convey the symptoms that we recognize or our minds are willing to share, but the information not shared could hold the key to all the manifestations of the illness or pain.

The answers to, "Why are you here?" are often superficial and reported in the well-learned style of progressive symptoms. "I've had headaches for a long time and now my eyes hurt." " I've always had low back pain so I'm used to that, but now my knees are swelling and sometimes I can hardly walk."

With each answer, I return to the timeline. Did the headaches start when you moved? Did you have an injury prior to the low back pain? Were you ever in an accident?

To some the questions may seem tedious and, certainly to those in the medical profession, this type of questioning would take too much time and not allow for the steady slow of the sick and dying. The questions are necessary. The true holistic practitioner knows that each person needs to be in charge of his or her own health and body. To be in charge requires knowledge, which requires memory and observation. When we learn how to ask ourselves the questions that lead to a beginning, we can eventually find the cause. When we take care of the cause, the symptoms disappear.

The body has a reason for being, part of which is providing a harbor for the soul. None of us as humans can fulfill our purpose without the body. The energy flowing through us changes and alerts us to imbalances, but we most often choose not to listen. We mask pain with drugs, cover wounds with ointments, repair teeth without questions, and remove organs without respect. What doctor whose Volvo had a check engine light on would remove the engine instead of finding the cause? Most of us take care of and understand our cars and computers better than we do our vital bodies. If you have rotated the tires on your SUV and not looked into how your shoes are affecting your balance or the wear and tear on your back, or if you've changed the oil every three thousand miles because you know it preserves the engine, but haven't paid attention to the oil balance, filters and lubrication of your body, you are one of the millions who believe your body's health and well-being is someone else's job. Are you mystified by computers because you believe they are some grand invention beyond your scope of understanding, or they're electronic monsters you have no use for so don't have to learn? Computers have viruses, worms, bad input, and they "crash." Diagnostics are done and "fixes" are implemented. You were the first computer, with input and output, read-only and random access memory, digital by nature, electronic by design. Demystify your body and take back the power inherently yours. Anatomy is not hard. Physiology is illogical to many, but sensible if you understand circles instead of lines. Pathology is understood by every mother who ever had a sick child.

When you begin to understand your physical being, you can also start to grasp the mental and spiritual sides of you. Together they form a triangle, the most powerful structure on Earth. The Pyramids remind us of this multidimensional truth. The mind, body, spirit connection is a balanced force and essential to all life. No one side of this triangle should be stronger than the other. When one takes precedence, the other sides have no choice but to collapse. If the spirit is all you concentrate on and you believe that will take care of everything in your life, your body will deteriorate and your mind will confuse you with its own short circuits. If you believe the mind is the only truly powerful part of you, your spirit may falter, and again your body may fail. If you concentrate only on your physical being, your mind and spirit can get confused. Even two out of three sides doesn't work. It takes three evenly balanced sides to make the triangle.

Most people interchange the words mind and brain, and then many just clump them together into "head." We have headaches, migraine headaches, sinus headaches, tension headaches, allergy headaches, and hangover headaches. The head becomes the scapegoat when, in fact, it's the mind and memory telling the brain to react so that we can determine the cause and alleviate it. The brain is the physical electronic connector box, with millions, perhaps trillions of interactive energy pulses and triggers guiding the body to reaction and function. The brain stem connects to our spinal column, which allows the impulses to travel to every organ, system and structure in the body. When the brain is declared dead, the energy that fuels life is shut off, and the soul/spirit within us leaves the harbor on another journey. Interesting that back surgery often fuses parts of the spine that normally would conduct this energy. Why do we believe this is a viable solution to back pain? Why don't we understand that not only can back pain be coming from spinal misalignment, mineral deficiency, polluted drinking and/or bathing water or a host of other causes, but also may be the body's way of telling us that one of our systems or organs normally innervated or "turned on" by that part of our spine is in trouble or needs attention? The system is out of balance, the mind troubled, the brain reactive and the gift of pain authorized.

When we approach our spiritual side, we often misinterpret this as religion or religious belief. We put our faith in God, pray and hope for relief or salvation. We're grateful when the pain is gone, or thankful for our child's return to health. Our mistake is the commingling of spirit with the institution of religion. In churches, we are once again told what to believe, how to believe, how to behave, how to judge. We're given textbooks, pamphlets, and catechisms with all the rules and laws of living translated and interpreted for us. If we believe in the Commandments, then we should know, as children do, that there are only a few rules to follow, otherwise we're free to do everything else. Even if we sometimes break those rules, if our intention was love and not fear, we will most likely be forgiven.

We need to understand that modern medicine came under the control of the church in the Middle Ages and remains under the university and church related laws of superiority and treatment. Doctors need not be creative in their treatment of patients or disease if they believe their cohorts and counterparts are the only viable source of information, and that the patient is not trained in medicine, therefore should be ignored. The church separated itself from the actual practice of physical medicine with the Renaissance, but maintains its position as the only authority on spiritual health regardless of denomination. This raises an imbalance with each individual's mind and body, as we are as unique as we are alike. The spiritual side of nature either stands in the forefront or takes a back seat, thus depleting the power of the pyramid or triangle and rendering us incapable of healing ourselves.

To know our spirit is to truly know God. There are no

thought processes, no arguments or dissertations, no textbooks or guides to Spirit. It is inherently ours and remains secluded or secretive only if we choose it to be. When we say a person is spirited or brings such spirit to a meeting or party, or is in good spirits, what we are recognizing is an energy that is always with us and asks only to be heard when necessary and felt every moment of every day. When we deny this, we systematically destroy the energy that helps to give us life. We feel depressed, low, attacked. We think of others as conspirators or begrudge their successes to justify our failures. We pray with our mouths instead of our hearts and desperately wait for answers to those prayers. When our energy is vibrant, in harmony, in the highest frequency, our spirits are high and we feel well. When we put those high spirits on the triangle with a strong and clear mind and a balanced body, we are healthy, whole human beings

CHAPTER II

Medicine in many Native American families means self-knowledge. The medicine people of the tribes were spiritual, but also herbalists who knew every aspect and purpose of God's weeds and plants. Great importance was attached to the Human connection to Earth, to nature, and to the Creator, and though anatomy was not a required course, medicine people intuitively and instinctively knew which herbs or plants affected which areas of the body and how that part of the body was supposed to work. They watched animals and plant life, the seasons, stars, and the moon and learned about cycles of change, digestion, blood circulation, life and death. By observing each other and the animals around them, they learned behaviors and personalities and attached names to their children based on their individual attributes. They understood the seasons and sat in medicine wheels that allowed the four directions of North, East, South and West to help guide them on their given paths.

Colors were given special meanings and their vibrations were felt through the senses of touch, vision and scent. Vegetables were given the highest honor by being called sisters of sustenance. Corn, beans and squash were family members devoted to cleansing and nourishing the body.

Water was medicine and they knew the water within their bodies needed to be clean. Sweat lodges to release impurities from the body, preceded by fasting and followed by a plunge in the river, were sacred healing rituals that ensured strength and long life.

European doctors, mostly from France, Italy and Germany, and the Arab physicians from Egypt practiced and tried to perfect surgical techniques and the science of discovery through analysis. The Greeks, of course, were considered the originators of medicine with people like Hippocrates and Galen, but they were replacements for the first healers, mostly women, who were naturalists and herbalists, astrologers and aromatherapists. These early practitioners were later labeled occultists and the churches of Italy put a stop to their practices. The monks became the keepers of the herbs, the original pharmacists, and any writings on alternative therapies were destroyed or hidden. These alternatives, as they are labeled today, were actually the mainstream of medicine, and many a prominent physician studied diet, nutrition and herbs before concentrating or specializing in a more accepted field.

Churches were the first hospitals for people who couldn't afford a personal physician or for needy travelers, and Priests were considered doctors. They often tended to royalty or the ruling class until they were stopped from performing surgery by practicing surgeons. Eventually, they concentrated more on religious medicine and remain the self-proclaimed authorities on spirit.

Inventions like the microscope furthered research into the microorganisms of the body, and much later led to inoculations for typhoid, smallpox and later polio, to name a few. Of course, these discoveries were important in understanding the body's defenses, but unfortunately, the science of medicine became more science than practice and the patients became secondary to research.

Alternative therapies took a back seat, but often were exactly as they were labeled- an alternative to the medicate or operate theories. More and more people today are turning to these therapies for pain management, stress reduction, and anything else the medical establishment doesn't, can't or won't provide.

The most common therapies or most familiar are those that deal directly with the body, such as massage, shiatsu, acupuncture and reflexology. Iridology, kinesiology, cranial-sacral and aromatherapy are lesser known or understood. Yoga, tai chi, hypnosis and energy medicine are more concerned with energy and the mind. In holistic health, these therapies are known as modalities. Much like the specialties of modern medicine, they need to be understood for their benefits, but none of them is the one answer anyone is looking for. Just as the general practitioner has all but disappeared from western medicine so, too, has the holistic practitioner.

When we first begin institutionalized learning about the body we treat it like tinker toys or erector sets. Each part is separate from the other and then joined by some kind of connector. We can take it apart and put it back together again, jiggle the skeleton in the corner and know it won't break, and see the wonders of reproduction in plastic models. We see ourselves as marvelous machines with many parts that form the whole, but we never truly understand our wholeness. The closest we get is knowing the song about which bones are connected to each other. If we've remembered all the words, when the song is done, we have a skeleton. Of course, the song doesn't tell us there are 26 bones in the feet or 27 in the hands or that the backbone is divided into cervical, thoracic and lumbar vertebrae. We know our pelvic girdle as either hips or no hips and that a shinbone is on the front of the leg because we kick people there. After a trip to the dentist, we may know about the temporal mandible joint that now causes our jaws to hurt, and we hear a little about the sacrum after we lift something heavy.

We do a little better with muscles because they're more visible and can serve our egos and vanity when in good condition. We build up our biceps and triceps, and call the abdominals, six-packs. We recognize tension in the neck and shoulders and are wise enough sometimes to stretch our quads or hamstrings before jogging. We treat what we believe to be muscle pain with salves, aspirin and ice, but we don't know what muscles eat or how they're made or where they actually connect. What is a sprained ankle? Why does tennis elbow hurt when you're not playing tennis? And why does it seem like everyone has to have shoulder surgery? When your back hurts, is it the bones, the muscles or the nerves? When you can't breathe, is it your lungs, your muscles, your spine or your diaphragm?

The nervous system can be more difficult because we can't see nerves. They're buried somewhere in our mass and when we're stressed, they act up. Stress in itself is bothersome and a cop-out. We need stress to survive. Our adrenals sit right above our kidneys and are always ready to fight or run. They also get tired when not nourished or allowed the healing time sleep provides, so any stress becomes more difficult to endure. The most stress anyone has ever gone through and we all have in common is being born. Most of us cried, but we got through it. As long as we were fed, the stress didn't bother us. What do nerves live on? Why do we use the word nerve to symbolize courage or audacity and still take drugs because "our nerves are on edge," or we have a nervous headache, worse yet, a breakdown?

The circulatory system seems to many the easiest to understand. After all, blood runs in our veins and when we're wounded, we bleed. Blood is red and we can see it, sometimes taste it. We know it's supposed to cover every inch of our bodies and we can donate it because it will replenish itself. We know we have blood relatives and have heard of those called bleeding hearts. We know some things may cause heart attacks or strokes and this, too, has something to do with our blood. In the fifties, we had iron-poor blood and now we have iron poisoning. If we have red blood cells and white blood cells, why isn't blood pink? Why are blood tests so important in diagnosing illness? Why do we say our blood turns cold when we're afraid, and yet we're warm-blooded mammals? Why is it that some see the bloodline as so important and place people into classified boxes according to their heritage?

The endocrine system can be more difficult than the nervous system. This one has been kept a mystery, and in modern medicine, there's a good reason. There are more drugs provided for an imbalance in this system than for any other. There are more surgeries done on women because of this imbalance than any other surgery. Keep it a mystery and keep the new house. Do a hysterectomy, put the woman on hormone replacement therapy, watch her thyroid because it's going to fail, then give her blood pressure medication, cut out the supposedly unimportant gall bladder, squeeze her mammary glands every year, send her to a psychotherapist when she's depressed, add Prozac or Zoloft to make her think she feels better, then treat her for liver disease and heart problems when she gets a little older.

The pituitary, hypothalamus, thymus, adrenals and thyroid are all a part of this system and need water, nourishment and balance to work as a team. They manage our emotions, our hormonal vicissitudes, our temperature, our moods, our secretions and excretions. They work with specific organs to regulate their functions and give us the keys to survival. If your thyroid is out of balance, is it because your adrenals are exhausted? Is your neck in proper alignment to innervate the thyroid? Is your thyroid acting as your "third ovary" because of imbalances elsewhere?

We know the heart pumps blood and the lungs give us air, but what does the liver do? Why is liver cancer so prevalent, and why does it seem that colon cancer occurs simultaneously? The word liver should give you a clue to its importance. Remove the letter "r" and know that you need this organ to live. It has more than five hundred jobs, but maybe the most important one to know right now is its role as the master filter. Nothing gets past the liver. Picture all the food, wine, candy and polluted water you've ever ingested going through this organ in one form or another. Picture minerals breaking down and depositing themselves in the liver because we didn't have a balanced diet and toxified ourselves with heavy metals. Imagine fats forming at the top of a saucepan filled with greasy meat and picture those same fats surrounding the liver. Maybe most importantly, look at the chemicals contained in your food and the number of pharmaceutical drugs you're taking. Where do you think they go? We don't flush all of these things out of our systems every day. Our tissues and organs, especially the liver, colon, and lungs, hold onto them just like the filter in your home furnace.

We need to know and understand this lively organ. We need to feel its energy and recognize its vibration. It holds our anger because it doesn't know how to filter anything so negative. It tries hard to clean our blood and help to provide oxygenated blood to the heart and lungs. It doesn't like acid, but disagrees more with antacids, and it does have a close relationship to the gall bladder, though modern medicine would have us believe otherwise. It helps to break down sugars so we can properly digest our food, and through the blood, provide nourishment for every cell. It absorbs alcohol and can contain stones much like the gallbladder or kidneys. Iron deficiency anemia, hepatitis, leukemia, and a host of other illnesses would not exist if we took proper care of the liver.

The pancreas and spleen are also an interesting pair. God put them on the left side of our bodies, right above the stomach, so they could take in and handle the sweetness of sugar and of life, and allow our immune system to still stay strong. Too much sweetness, too much stress, not enough liver function, a weakened spleen, and we have one of our most common ailments, diabetes.

The stomach is a friend to a few, an enemy to many, and is

not the round protrusion of fat and intestinal bloating that many refer to. It connects the esophagus in your throat to the intestinal tract at the other end, with the diaphragm in between. It contains acid and enzymes to help us digest food and actually does a little "chewing" to help move the food along. It shouldn't be very big, the size of your fist is about right, and it doesn't need the amount of food we try to stuff into it. Do you wonder why we're given antacids for digestive problems when it's acid that helps digestion? And how absurd, actually dangerous, is it that antacid companies are now targeting children's stomachs?

And then there are the intestines, large and small, and something called a colon that every doctor is sure has polyps. Five regular size meals are all the intestines should hold. This means you need to be getting rid of some of that stored waste about thirty to forty minutes after every meal. The colon is a hydrating, mucosal organ that expands with water intake and essentially dehydrates itself to expand and lubricate the fiber-containing waste material from our food. It has ridges and a muscular movement to push debris out of our bodies. When we over eat, it expands and distends and inflames, sometimes becoming permanently disfigured. When we don't drink water or substitute soda, coffee, tea and wine, the colon fills with gases from the rotten food and may even leak those gases back into our systems. It is the most important of our organs physiologically, and together with the liver, can either sustain or destroy our lives. When we can't move our bowels, we shoot water into our colon hoping that this form of hydration will do the trick. Or we take drugs that cause the nervous system to trigger movement and force the waste materials through the colon. When the colon is sick, the whole body is sick, so why do we poke and prod and then remove it piece by piece? Why do we believe its only job is to remove waste so a bag will do? Every single disease has its start in the colon. It seems doctors should have maintained their interest in nutrition and diet to do the most for their patients, rather than concentrating on the more lucrative specialty of surgery.

Let us not forget the skin, the largest organ in the body. Regardless of color, it is the most visible and maybe the most misunderstood. We have a basic understanding that it needs to be kept clean, not only for appearance, but also because something called germs and bacteria may reside on it. Some people cover the visible parts with lotions and oils hoping to bring out the luster or smoothness. Others spend their lives itching and scratching, or hiding as much of it as possible. We know we can get skin cancer and believe it comes from the sun. If you learn nothing else, learn this. Skin cancer does not come from the sun. The skin absorbs everything we touch, including our bath and shower water, and is hydrated and cleansed from within. When water was healthy, food was grown in healthy soil and the air was clean, there was no skin cancer. If the liver is full of sludge, the colon stagnant and the water full of chlorine or its by-products, there's a good chance the UV rays from the sun will signal us with cancerous growths. Surgery, again, is the course of action. When was the last time an oncologist or dermatologist asked you about the water in your home or the water you drink or your bowel movements or your birthplace before cutting your skin to remove a tumor?

Even a rudimentary understanding of the body can help us get on the path to self-health and healing. We don't need to know all the ins and outs or even pretend that we do. The body is physical, biochemical and mechanical, but it is also electrical. If we can "tune in" to our energy, feel it, be in harmony with it, the body, mind and spirit will come together to give us the answers and show us the way to balance. To better understand this energy, consider what we already know. The Earth has a North and a South Pole, polarity, positive and negative charges. Beneath the Earth's surface are Tectonic plates, magnets of enormous size that constantly shift and reposition. The elements of the Earth are those you remember from Chemistry class in high school. Each one has an atomic number, each a positive or negative charge. Opposites attract and likes repel. As the plates move, the minerals move. Lightning is, in basic terms, electricity from the atmosphere, striking the Earth hundreds of times a day, ionizing the air and water while it recharges the surface.

Now put us in the middle. We're made of the same minerals and the energy of the Earth flows through us giving us life, or what in Chinese medicine is referred to as Chi. This electric flow is constant and causes an electro-magnetic field around us. From our feet, if we're standing, or from our sacrum while sitting, the energy flows through and around our bodies, from Earth to Heaven and back. We are conduits, conductors of this force and intended to be vibrant, clear light.

Look at a healthy, newborn baby, from healthy parents, after it has "connected" to being a human being. Its skin is radiant, almost translucent, and its fingernails are pink and smooth. No dark circles or bags under the eyes. No pock marks or pimples or morning backaches or sinus headaches or swollen feet. Then we feed it. We give it sugar water and breast milk filled with chemicals. We bathe it in polluted tap water and parade it around grocery stores and chlorinated swimming pools. We cover it with creams and lotions so its skin can absorb every chemical. When he or she gets older, we send her to school with peanut butter sandwiches on white bread, cow's milk or soda, and hydrogenated potatoes. By now she's had several inoculations and ingested liters and pounds of unhealthy substances. She's sick, out of balance, and in her own way tries desperately to tell us. She's angry all the time, or moody, or doesn't pay attention or listen. We put her on antibiotics because we need to go to work, and feed her cough medicine and allergy medications because her nose is always running and she never gets rid of her cough. She urinates and defecates and all the chemicals and medications go back into the water system to be treated with chlorine and other chemicals so that drinking water, the water she'll get from the drinking fountain or your tap, will be governmentally safe. When she won't drink water because she intuitively knows the chlorine is bad for her, we train her to drink soda or sugary fruit juices. Her liver is already in trouble and her colon is becoming a sludge-filled, galvanized pipe. Because hormonal by-products are released in the water system and chickens and cows are fed hormones to fetch a better price, she's eight or nine years old and begins to menstruate. The cramping is horrendous and painful, so we give her water pills and pain relievers. Her skin is full of eruptions and she often gets headaches. She oversleeps or wakes up grumpy. She looks to music to soothe her soul and finds the vibrations of anger, lust, and hatred. From fear of rejection, she spends hours every day putting on make-up and doing her hair. The mall is her home as she worriedly tries to fit in with every wardrobe purchase. Her heart aches. And she's only twelve years old.

She grows a little more, gets depressed, or so we're told, and starts a regimen of antidepressants and birth control pills. Illegal drugs make her feel better than prescriptions, and alcohol helps to remove the memory of a childhood she's already lost and doesn't want to remember. She finds someone she believes she loves. He's on antidepressants, too, and has been treated for venereal disease because sex with anyone was always okay. He's a boy, after all, and like his father before him, he's learned to act out his fear with virility and apathy. He's angry, though he doesn't always know why, and he's not sure he'll ever be "man enough" to take on the world as he's been told he should. He eats super-sized meals of hormonal beef and pizza, doesn't pay attention to the parts of him that hurt, nor believes he has to. His health is someone else's job. He'll put his trust in his sexual prowess, try to land an athletic scholarship, and consider suicide when he doesn't make the grade. He'll have prostate cancer before he's sixty, diverticulosis that he treats with more drugs, and worry about heart attacks his entire life. The two of them have a lot in common. Together they'll make babies and a life together. And so the cycle continues.

Can we change this cycle? Absolutely. We were meant to heal ourselves and to know when to look for outside help and where to find it

CHAPTER III

Alternative medicine modalities have been in existence since the beginning of time. Reflexology is perhaps one of the oldest practices recognized in the United States that is the closest to a holistic approach to the body. It is the art and science of applying on and off pressure to the feet and hands in a manner that affects every organ and system. Because we are upright and energy travels through us, and because we live in a gravitational atmosphere, everything goes to our feet. Circulation allows nutrients and oxygen to go to our toes and back, but what also happens is sediment from the debris in our bodies that the blood, liver and lymphatic system can't handle. Can you see it in an X-ray or a CT scan? No. This isn't physical debris like garbage on the street. This is energetic trash that can form uric crystals and block energy from its due course. If we can't receive the energy from the earth, or release the debris, all of our organs and systems begin to suffer. Because we rely on this energy, our bodies feel uncomfortable and depleted without it. When we're uncomfortable, we are in dis-ease. If we don't pay attention to pain or discomfort or disease, we fall into a worsened state of actual disease that eventually leads to death.

In many Native American tribes, death is simply part of the cycle of life. Leaves die and come back in the spring to remind us that life will always continue. Though losses of life are mourned, the life energy that being brought to Earth is also celebrated and revered. Their spirit energy is considered eternal and their transition from life to death is a transformation and journey to another cycle. If we think multi-dimensionally, we can understand this transition as not one that takes us to a Heaven or a Hell, but rather one that allows all time and place to be seen and experienced simultaneously, with only the depth or denseness of the experience being different. What is already was, and whatever is to be, is already. Erase the timeline we've all learned to live and die by and replace it with a circle, no beginning and no end. Now go one step further and spiral that circle into many other circles with some parts of the circle touching the others at different times as they continuously spin. The past is now. Ancestors send us thought patterns and emotions as they dream of the future. Great grandchildren listen to our wisdom as they relate to the past. We are given the opportunity to recreate our lives and ourselves every day. Is it any wonder with all the hate, crime, violence and pollution that we crave recreation so earnestly? Heaven is right here, and so is Hell, or whatever you believe in. By living every moment without fear, but rather with love, we create our lives and recreate them. When we destroy the energy of our bodies, we cease to exist as humans. Does that mean we re-incarnate? If you believe that to be so, then so it is. Does that mean we follow a light to Heaven where we're judged for entry? If you believe it to be, then so it is; however, get rid of the judgment part. Unconditional love means just that. Judgment comes from fear and fear cannot exist where there is love. Everything around us has energy and life. Everything is somewhere on the circles, sometimes touching us, influencing us, reminding us, teaching us. The tiniest particle, the smallest blade of grass is as important as we are because it was created, not by man, but by the energy that creates life. It was created by God and we recreate it.

We also create dis-ease. If we can create it, we can re-create it and change its path. We can reverse the energy of the circle of disease until we're back in our purest form. Homeopathy is the science that attempts to do this through naturopathic formulas.

Reflexology, done correctly, can open the energy path through the feet and hands and allow the debris to dissipate and disappear.

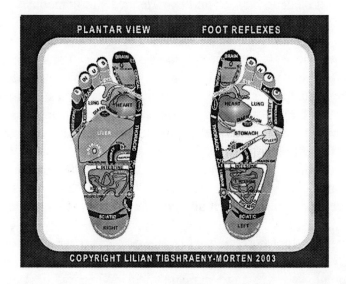

There are several methods of reflexology, the most trusted being the Eunice Ingham approach. Introduced to the United States in 1938, Ingham chronicled hundreds of patients and developed a foot chart that maps the zones and path of energy to every organ and system. Lillian Tibshraeny-Morton incorporates both the Ingham approach and the connection to Chinese meridians. By using a "thumb-walking" method of on and off pressure, the practitioner can release the body's energy within the context of the pulse. This method not only physically eliminates uric crystals that settle in the feet, but also attunes the body's natural rhythm of electro-magnetic energy.

The chart is a reflection of our anatomy and the 10 zones travel the length of us from head to toe. If you look at someone's feet facing you, the charts will make perfect sense. The tops of the toes correspond to the head and brain; the spine has two curves and follows the inside curve of the foot from the large toe to the heel. The hands are a little more difficult to envision because the surface area is different and the fingers usually longer than the toes, but if you've ever seen someone rubbing their hands nervously before a speech, what you might have witnessed is hand reflexology helping them to relax and breathe as they reflexed the diaphragm.

Reflexology is taught in massage schools, but a certified reflexologist studies and practices for hundreds of hours before finally taking an extensive written and practical exam. Beware of those who refer to this method as foot massage. It is not. Varying degrees of pressure and focused communication with the client is fundamental. When done correctly, the goal is relaxation, and when the body is no longer fighting to rid itself of waste in the vital area that channels energy, it can relax.

Reflexologists don't diagnose or prescribe, but the benefit of this modality is more than relaxation. If an area or zone of your foot is particularly tender, a good practitioner may ask you questions about your digestion or elimination. If a specific reflex point is sensitive, he or she may ask other questions regarding diet or sleep habits or anything that may help you to find the cause of your dis-ease. Sessions should be fifty minutes to an hour, but one of the keys to success using reflexology is consistency and change.

Reflexology is most often done in a reflexology chair, a chaise lounge that lets you lie back and elevates your feet for the therapist. You are fully clothed, which often makes this therapy more desirable for those in a hurry or those afraid of their bodies. Most of the time no oils or lotions are used, though many Reflexologists are being trained in the powerful effects of therapeutic essential oils and will apply these to reflex points on the feet. Your therapist will be able to see your face and may converse with you about tenderness and pressure on your feet.

When you've determined that your feet are signaling a congested area such as the colon and you know your diet has been unbalanced, it's time to take action. If your lung area is congested, you could be holding onto grief, smoking too much, or in need of an air filtration system in your home. If your spinal reflexes are consistently tender, you may need to stretch more or get arch supports for your shoes or drink more water. As the tenderness in these areas subsides in subsequent sessions, you may find yourself feeling more balanced with more energy. Reflexology has accomplished its goal, because when you feel better, you're more relaxed, and that's one of the results the therapist was trying to accomplish.

Massage is another touch modality that varies in reputation, has been abused by pleasure-seekers, and has several specialties attached to it. It's popular in health spas and resorts and is mostly performed by licensed massage therapists. Notice the word "therapist" versus masseuse or masseur. A licensed therapist has taken anywhere from 700 to one thousand hours or more of classroom instruction. The curriculum varies slightly from state to state, but in general covers anatomy, physiology, kinesiology, pathology, massage history, ethics, hygiene, hydrotherapy, some shiatsu and some reflexology. Many states require a license and most require National certification and continuing education to maintain it.

The art and science of massage was developed by a gymnast who recognized that exertion causes acids to build up in the muscles, and unless the muscles are stroked, kneaded, and stretched, the acid condition will not only cause pain, but will also impede nutrition and circulation. Increased circulation is only one benefit of therapeutic massage. Because circulation is increased and oxygenated blood is flowing to the heart, it can lower blood pressure. Joints need lubrication to work properly, and increased blood flow to the tendons and ligaments that attach muscle to bone and muscles to each other helps to keep the joints fluid and reduces inflammation. The lymphatic system lies just beneath the surface of the skin and is the "garbage collector." It doesn't have a pump like the circulatory system does, so the only way it can maintain a flow is through muscle contraction and movement. Massage increases this flow and helps to rid the body of anything the lymphatic system has attacked as foreign.

The emotional benefits of massage are also important. Human beings need to be touched, not in an offensive way, but in a caring and loving way. Babies and animals respond immediately to back or foot massage as a signal from the giver that we care and want them to know we're here for them.

When massage first came to America, it was almost immediately cheapened to a pleasure-seeking practice in brothels and whorehouses. With that reputation came the fear from many that this gentle and loving practice was nothing more than sexual distraction and should be avoided. Thankfully, therapists continued to educate the public on the benefits and procedures of massage. The ignorant still scoff and the fearful stay untouched, but spas, resorts and private practices are teeming with those who know it's healthy, safe, and performed ethically.

Doctors, nurses and other health care professionals have started accepting massage as a piecemeal therapy for their patients. Therapists are asked to massage shoulders, knees and lower backs to help alleviate pain.

There are now a host of massage specialties, some viable, others grasping for some ethereal bond between the therapist and Heaven. Many therapists refer to themselves as "healers." The only one who can heal you is you. If you believe in God, He'll help you heal yourself. Those who refer to themselves as healers are often more attached to ego than spirit, and they clamor after every new approach to put it on their business cards.

The difference between therapeutic, relaxation, and deep tissue massage is or should be the amount of pressure imposed by the therapist and nothing else. Massage is inherently therapeutic as it helps the body to balance itself. When the body is balanced, it's relaxed. If the therapist has to exert more pressure, go deeper into the tissues, it's usually because the body, especially the muscles, are dehydrated or undernourished. The muscles have lost their flexibility and pulled the spine out of alignment. If the spine is not aligned, every muscle group will be taxed and will signal us with aches or cramping.

Hot oil massage is a gimmick that some believe feels better than cold lotion or massage cream. Hot stone massage does have benefits as stones retain minerals and our muscles need them; however, the absorption from the stones is minimal. Perhaps we've learned to dislike the cold instruments in doctor's offices and hospitals, so hot stones, hot oil and warm hands feel less threatening.

The proper way to receive a massage is without clothes. It's impossible for any therapist to feel tension or muscle congestion through synthetic clothing, and the receiver also needs to feel the massage strokes to not only signal the need for more pressure, but to enjoy the very human comfort of touch. Massage therapists are taught to deal with the delicate matter of nudity through proper draping. This means the only parts of the body exposed are the parts being worked on, and this is done in the most modest manner.

Therapists start you on your back or your stomach, depending on their preference. Some start with the head and face, others with the feet. It doesn't really matter which end they start with as long as the continuous flow of energy is clockwise and toward the heart. Every part of the body except the genitals and female breasts need to be massaged. Actually, the breasts would benefit greatly from therapeutic massage, but we are still too much of a misogynistic society to not objectify women. If your therapist skips your pectorals and abdomen because you are a female, fire them. If they don't do your gluts, meaning your buttocks, fire them.

The abdominal area is critical in massage therapy as the therapist can often feel congestion, swelling, masses or inflammation. The gall bladder and colon can signal acute problems so the therapist can refer you to the proper doctors.

Gluteus Maximus, Medius and Minimus are the thickest muscles we have and overlap each other to give us a behind and balance and movement. They are attached to the hips and the back and need special attention because of their mass.

Energetically, it is unhealthy to have a massage up to but not including your abdomen, and then up your legs but not including your gluts. All the energy is pushed to the center and left there to fend for itself. Massage should be full body, and when it's full body, that means everything but the most private parts.

Music is used in both reflexology and massage to help the client relax. Countless research has been done on tonal awakening, harmonious tuning, and the benefits of vibrational energy on helping the body to come back into balance. We are, after all, full of various vibrations and frequencies. We are energy. We are electric. From the moment the umbilical cord is cut and we are separated from Mother and from God, we begin to resonate as human beings. As the blood begins to flow independently and oxygen is breathed into the lungs, our energy centers, or chakras, begin to open.

To simplify energy and electricity draw a straight line and from the beginning point on that line draw an arch to the halfway point. From there draw another arch beneath the line to the end. This is a sine wave. Electricity runs negative to positive and the sine wave shows the number of proportional oscillations per second. Frequency is the measurement of these oscillations. Color has different frequencies. Your radio has different frequencies. Our bodies have various frequencies. Death occurs at 25 Megahertz, so we obviously want to keep our frequencies high. Every organ and system has its own frequency of optimal health. The healthier it is, the greater the vibration. The electro-magnetic force that surrounds the Earth and us most definitely helps us to live.

Each chakra center is a different frequency, the base or root chakra is the lowest, and the crown chakra is the highest. The frequency of our base chakra is basically the same as the color red. This chakra is the first to open as blood streams through our veins and arteries. It sends oxygen and nutrients to all of our systems and organs and essentially tells them, "Wake up! We're on our own!" Our vibration increases and the next chakra to open is in the digestive area. If we don't eat within seven or eight hours, we will die, so this chakra vibrates furiously to let us know we're hungry.

Because we are now human beings with a will to survive, the next chakra to open is the solar plexus. Its frequency is yellow and we call this our fear center. It's directly complementary to the root or base chakra as its activation tells us what we need to survive. Yellow and red make the color orange. We fear dying from starvation so our yellow chakra is open wide.

As our subconscious awakens and our souls realize we are now human, the heart chakra opens and fills with vibrational love. We root around hoping to find the one who loves us and will feed us. We have no judgment or fear. At this point we are unconditionally, loving human beings. If the digestive chakra tells us there's no food, our communication chakra at the throat opens and we let this vibratory color of blue let everyone know we're hungry.

For now, the first five of seven chakras are awake and our physical bodies are becoming attuned to our walk on Earth. The sixth chakra won't be fully open for a while. It needs that energy that comes from experience and discernment. It is the combined frequencies of our base or survival chakra and our communication center, red and blue. This purple frequency will be dimmed in many as they continue to grow physically, but not mentally or spiritually. This is also what many refer to as "the third eye," the intuitive center. Only through the experience of living from the heart, striving for unconditional love, and allowing the whispers from our souls, will this chakra ever be vibrant purple.

We get some help from above, of course. The seventh, or crown chakra, is white. White is the frequency of all colors, and is also the beginning of no color at all. This chakra is the highest frequency and we'll spend our lifetimes trying to raise all of our vibrations to this level.

Imagine you are a multi-sided crystal and the white light is shining through you. When the sun shines through an unblemished, unblocked crystal, we see a rainbow. If we put black tape over any facet, the rainbow changes. Some of the colors will be missing. If we continue to tape, the rainbow will completely disappear.

Our chakras are the same colors as a rainbow, that beautiful arch formed from water and light. We are 80% water, and as the light from above shines through us, we should reflect all of these colors. Physical trauma, emotional imbalance, spiritual neglect, negative energy, judgment, fear, anger, hate – any vibration that doesn't resonate with unconditional love of self and others, will essentially put a black veil over that facet of our lives.

Auras are essentially the outward emanations of this chakra energy, which many believe also show our spirit guides or teachers when photographed with a Holographic camera. Just as atoms are not the perfect circles, we learned about in chemistry and physics classes, neither is our chakra energy perfect and stable. Our electrons shoot out in all directions, and when healthy, are very active. We can affect the energy of others by a mere glance, a touch, even a thought.

You stop at a traffic light and think about work or school, or remember the anger you had yesterday or last year. You glance at the car opposite yours, and in an instant, transfer that energy to the other driver. He drives away and suddenly begins to feel angry and doesn't know why. Much later, the angry energy still brewing within, another driver cuts him off, and he finds himself raging, ready to fight, even to kill.

You walk into a restaurant feeling shy and vulnerable because you're by yourself. Your energy is defensive, afraid, and you respond to the waitress rudely. When she returns with your meal she, too, is rude, though she doesn't consciously know why, and the two of you continue the scenario throughout the meal.

You go to a party feeling strong and positive. The first person you meet feels that energy and is immediately attracted to you. You spend the night sharing stories and laughter, and by the end of the evening, you both feel loved and supported.

Music can help clear some of the black tape. The vibrations from music have been shown to relax the body and the mind, often allowing us to get out of the physical and attune our minds and souls. If the vibration is too low or full of static, our frequencies are also static. If you've ever tried to tune a radio when there isn't clear reception, you'll recognize the sound and feeling of that static. Clear reception is the key. To absorb the energy from Heaven or above, our body, mind, and spirit have to be clear. Church choirs and "heavenly" music often put us in a higher vibration, a higher state of being. Rap music brings the vibrational levels very low, opening the survival chakra instead of the crown. The sounds of the forties and fifties were very mellow and resonated to the heart and digestive chakras. We wanted love, and we were at a point in our history when we were ready to take in and digest everything we could see or hear in the world. Elvis didn't resonate with many because rock and roll disrupted our basic mineral balance and made us feel nervous, disconnected.

The Bible tells stories of music soothing the hearts of men, as with David's harp and King Saul. When we create music, we are expressing our inner vibrations, our soul frequencies. Classical music climbs the scales and is often performed by orchestras. This allows for a variety of frequencies and may help to balance or soothe our minds. New Age music is known for its harmonics, and Native American music often resonates with drums and flutes. This music has been found to be the most therapeutic in overall body and mind relaxation. It may remind us of mother's heartbeat in the safety of the womb, or perhaps allows our souls to remember Earth's heartbeat when we first joined the human race.

Listen to the music in our world today.

Rebalancing the chakras takes more than a pendulum or a spinning hand. If we picture each chakra center as a water balloon, all lined up from bottom to top, they should all be equally filled, each allowing room for the other and all in balanced harmony. If we've decided that eating is our main reason for being here, our digestive chakra grows and fills with the energy of food. If we are so centered on eating as a "way of life," this orange balloon is going to overshadow our root chakra and our solar plexus. Our root chakra, the red balloon, will begin to feel crowded and squeezed, but since it is the first chakra and vibrates with the survival frequency, it panics and alerts the yellow, solar plexus. The fear center is now open and is also panicked. We've begun a vicious circle. The physical body will begin to deteriorate in the abdominal area as we continue stuffing it with food. The root chakra will cry out for survival and the reproductive organs associated with it will also be filled with static energy. Is it any wonder, given the music our children listen to today, that many are fearful, angry, overeaters, who believe sex is the key to life?

Our communication chakra, the blue vibration, is in our throat area. We communicate through words and sounds, harmonics that make us understood. Our primal scream is the yawn and many believe it is the same "scream" recognized throughout the animal kingdom by parents of any species. Just as penguins communicate through the most minute changes in vibration, so do we. As we learn to integrate our energy into words, our levels and intentions of communication change. We speak according to our teachers and the words we create also create our actions. The blue chakra is open long before the higher chakra of wisdom, perhaps as a lifelong lesson to be aware of our words and that all vibrations emitted from us are not only important, but also have the potential to change our paths and the paths of others.

Listen to your own speech patterns, those on television and in song lyrics. "Trash" is being created everywhere. Many people don't even know how to speak without sexual utterances and damning interjections.

Our vocal chords should be our harp strings, and the melodies should be coming from the heart and the soul. Because our minds listen to everything we do and say, we are "teaching" our minds anger, hatred, disease, and ultimately death. We say to our children, "I'll kill you if you do that again." We tell each other to "Go to Hell," along with many other expletives. Often we blame our words on anger and then try to "take them back," as if the vibrational energy was something able to be caught, bottled or erased. Every time we say we're sick, we will be. Whenever we declare ourselves as "half dead," we will be. When we say to another, "You look awful," they will. How many times have you said, "I wish I was dead?"

Balancing our energy can be a big job. Many people believe they are on a "spiritual" path, that they are closer to God and doing everything they can to raise their vibration to the divine. Unfortunately, the higher chakras are still balloons. If we constantly fill our heads, minds and senses with what we believe to be spiritual endeavors, we crowd the purple chakra and deplete the others. The purple chakra is different from red, orange, or yellow. When crowded, it shrinks. The energy of wisdom and experience is not in balance with the physical experience of being human. Instead of crying out in strength, it secludes itself, and leaves many wondering why? They ask why they can't feel what someone else does, or hear that inner voice as others do when they've worked so hard to walk the spiritual path. The only way to truly open this chakra is to "walk your talk." Share your spirit. Don't be afraid of loving with all of your heart. Take in and digest the fears of others, then send those fears to the ground. Embrace your spirit, and then embrace the people next to you. They, too, are on a path, and their circles of energy and life touch yours. Feel their pain. Feel their longing. Feel their love. Then open all of your chakras to the experience of life. When they are all in balance, the wisdom chakra will open and harmonize.

How does this energy travel our physical bodies? Ah, the nervous system again. It controls and coordinates all organs and structures in the body. Your house or apartment has many wires running it through it to turn lights off and control or maintain thermostats for furnaces and blowers, allow appliances to operate, even the doorbell to ring. All of these wires go to a fuse or circuit breaker box, and from there to a utility grid.

Your spine and nervous system are similar to this network of energy. Each spinal nerve controls or helps to control a part of your body. Misalignment of any of the vertebrae or discs along the spine may cause irritation to the nervous system.

If you are sitting, you are most likely putting direct pressure on your sacrum, and related pressure on other parts of your back. This is okay, as your spine was intended to support you while sitting or standing. If you're experiencing low back pain, it could be there is misalignment of the spine at the sacral area, which could also affect the hips. Or, maybe you've been walking barefoot and caused your hips to go out of alignment. Your sacrum will signal you.

If your knees are also hurting, it could be that Lumbar 3, which innervates the knee area, is the point of misalignment, or again, your hips are causing your knees to compensate so you stay upright, and L3 is alerting you.

God created chiropractors to help us learn and deal with these misalignments. They're not bone doctors or back crackers. They specialize in the nervous system, particularly spinal nerves, and are well trained in the consequences of nerve impingement, disc sublaxation, herniation and a host of other problems associated not only with back pain, but also with imbalances in any organ or system. The best ones are holistic in their approach and will help you to learn about the relationship between your spine and the troubled organ or system. Alignment in the spinal area will often help the body to "heal" itself energetically.

Follow your spine from bottom to top. The coccyx, or tailbone, then the sacrum, five lumbar, twelve thoracics and seven cervicals. That bump at the base of your neck is cervical or C7. C1 affects the brain supply to the head, the pituitary gland, the brain, the inner and middle ear. Earaches are often C1.

C2 affects the eyes, sinuses, tongue, and forehead, C3 the teeth, and C4 the Eustachian tube. How many babies have tubes surgically inserted to allow drainage from the sinuses through the Eustachian tube? Did anyone check their necks or backs?

C6 affects neck muscles, shoulders and tonsils, and C7 the thyroid gland. Whiplash, poor bed pillows, and poor posture in general can cause the cervicals to become misaligned.

Thoracic or T1 affects your hands, wrists and fingers. T2 the heart and coronary arteries, and T3 the lungs, bronchial tubes, and breasts. I know what you're thinking and you're right. Carpel tunnel syndrome may be coming from misalignment of the neck and upper back, caused by sitting at a computer improperly or sleeping on the couch in an awkward position. Worse than that, thyroid medication may be prescribed because of simple misalignment of C7 causing a thyroid test to register weakness.

T4 is your gall bladder, T5 the liver and general circulation. T6 handles your stomach, T7 the pancreas and T8 the spleen. Your adrenals and kidneys are T9 through T11 and your small intestine is plugged in at T12.

Your large intestine, appendix, abdomen, upper legs, prostate gland, uterus, bladder, knees, lower back and feet, are all turned on by L1 through L5, the largest bones in the spine.

Acne, pimples and eczema can come from T11. Hives and allergies can come from T9 and asthma can originate from problems with T1.

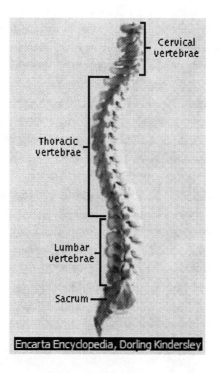

Encarta Encyclopedia, Dorling Kindersley

Our backs hold us upright and allow us to move forward. We carry our past with us always. Unresolved problems from childhood or a failed marriage, an abusive father or overbearing mother, all show up in the spine because we use our bodies to express our emotions. We cower when we're afraid of authority, or hold back tears when we're told to be tough. We slouch when our self-esteem is low and sleep on our stomachs when we feel too vulnerable. We don't physically stretch to unlock this energy, nor do we stretch our souls to release it. The muscles get pulled and twisted because the bones are crooked, and the nervous system ends up as tangled as Christmas lights from the bottom of the box.

Psychotherapists will sometimes tell people they need to "get in touch" with their anger, assuming reliving the past will somehow eradicate it. If you had two buckets, one filled with sticky, awful stuff, and one filled with soft, cushy stuff, which would you rather be "in touch with?" Love is the soft stuff, and love starts with us. Look in the mirror and tell that best friend looking back at you, "I love you." Forgive yourself. Let go of the anger over the past and recognize that everything that's ever happened to you is a gift. There are no wrong turns and this is not a rehearsal. This journey we call life is the destination and we need to embrace every moment. You chose to be here. You chose your parents and your hometown. You also chose the lessons you came here to learn. You have an agreement with God and your soul to learn from every encounter, every perceived mistake, every hurt and every fear. Perhaps you're here to learn forgiveness. Maybe your lesson is humility or unconditional love. You likely chose to learn more than one special lesson and your life seems complicated with all the twists and turns. Remember that all roads lead to Heaven.

When we harbor anger, it's like a tattoo on our backs. It blocks life- giving energy and our bodies cry out in pain. The liver has to filter these emotions, as does the spleen and every tissue, so the middle of our backs constantly ache. If the middle is in trouble, so are both ends, the cervicals and the sacral area, because we're like suspension bridges and every bounce or sway directly affects the complementary angle. The neck and the lower back can react so violently that we're forced to stop our walk. The soul is the traffic cop and essentially tries to tell us that anger, fear, and resentment are not what we're here for, and if we continue to harbor them, we will feel dis-ease. Turn a deaf ear or mask the pain and other areas of the body will join in.

Animals can teach us a lot about the way we deal with emotions and pain. Each species has its own special traits, another gift to us as we do our earthwalk. Something as simple as a butterfly can help us learn that change is good, and need not be traumatic. They dance on flowers to remind us to do the same, to lighten up and enjoy the beauty of the world around us. In early Christianity, the butterfly was the symbol of the soul and to Native Americans, a symbol of change, joy and color.

Let go. Give up the past to whatever higher source you believe in. Trust in something or someone higher than yourself. To some this is referred to as faith. Here's a challenge. If you were a lone climber on a high, jagged mountain and suddenly slipped with only a rope to stop your fall, what would you do? It's dark, and cold, and you're afraid. You can't see anything and you feel your hands slipping as you try desperately to hold on. You pray for help, and to your amazement a voice answers. "Let go," the voice says, and you know in your heart it is God speaking. "But I can't," you answer. "I'll fall and be hurt, or worse, I'll be killed."

"Let go," the voice repeats lovingly.

"Please," you say. "Help me. I'm freezing and I don't want to fall."

What would you do?

The next morning hikers find you frozen, dangling from a rope, three short feet from the ground. Where was your trust? Where was your faith? What causes us to come into this world with unconditional love and faith, and then grow into fear, distrust and a sense that we are somehow in control? When the Bible says, "Come to me as little children," why when we become adults do we forget that inner child and pretend that we know more than our Creator does?

Your physical body will alarm you when your soul is unhappy. Your spine is an important key and paying attention to its messages can help you get back into balance. Instead of carrying what we perceive to be our unhappy childhood or some other disturbing moment from the past, we would be wise to let the past be behind us as it was meant to be and consider it a gift to help us on our journey. Chiropractic can align the energy, but we have to do the emotional, spiritual work of releasing the negative.

One modality that is now being more accepted as a viable alternative to drugs or surgery is hypnosis. We often think of this as the entertaining hypnotist who forces people to behave in ways they normally wouldn't, rather than a path to healing.

Native American Shamans believe that the mind is made up of at least three separate energies, the conscious, the subconscious, and the higher self, or unconscious, that encompasses the more powerful energy of the Creator. Shamanic trances will tap into the higher self to "see" the path of imbalance or the outcome of a series of events. The Shaman often chants or hums to clear any static energy. This releases the conscious mind from thought, and frees the unconscious from memory. This type of meditation or self-hypnosis has been used by various religions and belief systems for thousands of years and is often feared by those who live only in the conscious mind. Interestingly, it is churches who practice hypnosis and chanting publicly and deliberately, mandating certain prayers and songs to essentially hypnotize congregations into obedience of their tenets. Though many of these rituals appear to propel us closer to the Divine, the subliminal messages are more often fear, judgment, and superiority raising conflict in physical and mental energies. The unconscious mind retains these suggestions and we often see the physical manifestations in knee problems, memory inconsistencies, weight gain and migraines. The emotional manifestations can be depression, aggressive behavior and manic-depressive schizophrenia.

The clinical hypnotist will use hypnosis to clear the path to the subconscious and attempt to have the client release the memories or imprints that are causing imbalance. One of the problems with this modality is its use as the be-all-end-all course of action, rather than a complementary practice of unconscious awakening.

Another form of hypnosis is past-life regression. A practitioner facilitates the client's journey into the sub-conscious past and helps them to realize aspects of their "past lives." This modality relies on the belief that we have lived many times before, rather than the alternative belief that all lives are concurrent and therefore in the present. The most prevalent belief is that we have but one life with a beginning and an end on a predetermined and unalterable timeline so there can be no past lives. Whatever the belief, the subconscious and unconscious minds can provide more keys to our physical, mental and spiritual health and we need to respect their place in our overall balance.

The one modality that is perhaps most misunderstood, takes the longest to learn, is the least practiced and is becoming the most abused is iridology. Poets have long written about the eyes as being the windows of the soul. Iridology is the practice of "reading" the eyes, particularly the iris, to determine weaknesses in organ and body systems and essentially map the course of illness, injury and disease. The eyes are aqueous, dependant on water, and conduct millions of electrical stimuli. We look, but don't see, and sometimes see without looking. Our eyes participate in images recorded from the conscious, subconscious and the unconscious. The iris is one of the most complex tissue structures in the body with thousands of fine, white fibers organized into three layers. The eyes are extensions of the brain, including the emotional brain. Dilation and contraction of the pupils indicate excitement, tenseness or drug induced chemical reactions. Though every iris is unique, the pattern of information recorded is identical in every person. We can correlate the physical anatomy to every part of the eye, and can analyze the "reflexive" energy displayed in the iris.

A physician who grew up in the 1800's caught an owl in his garden at the age of eleven. In the struggle, the owl's leg was accidentally broken. The boy could see a straight, black line emerging in the iris of the owl, and kept special records of the changes in this line as he bandaged the leg and nursed the owl back to health. The black line changed to white and crooked lines as the leg healed.

Iridologists map the iris in a circle and use the hour positions of a clock with ten subdivisions between each hour. The right iris reflects the right side of the body and the left iris reflects the left side. Your liver and gall bladder are on your right side, so your right eye will show weakness, disease, trauma or surgery. Your pancreas, spleen and heart are on your left side, so the left iris reflects imbalances in these organs.

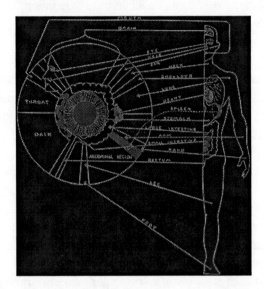

Iridology doesn't diagnose disease. The analysis of the iris can reveal inflammation, toxicity, and a pattern of repair or disintegration, but it should never be used as a diagnostic tool. Every individual's history and presence is different, and every individual manifests disease differently depending on all the variables that cause our imbalance. A line at one juncture in the eye could indicate a weakness in the heart, but you may develop heartburn, while I may develop heart disease. Diagnosis by definition is the categorizing of symptoms into specific names. Iridology doesn't see symptoms, but rather tissue conditions that usually reveal themselves long before symptoms occur.

Because the path of disease can be a long one, beginning with imbalances and progressing through discomfort, dis-ease, and finally disease, iridology becomes invaluable in seeing the beginning of these pathologies long before any recognized symptoms show themselves.

Iridology is one of the most holistic modalities available, but is also the most abused. Those who believe in the dollar more than the purpose have purchased cameras and computers to photograph the iris, and subsequently, suggest supplements to eradicate weaknesses, yet their training in holistic practices is limited or non-existent and the consumer/client is often left again with a drawer or cupboard full of herbs, vitamins and miracle cures that the camera operator has suggested. The cameras and computers are valuable tools, but only in the hands of those who have truly studied this complex art and science and who also have a thorough knowledge of the body, mind and spirit.

If we straighten the iris and lay it side-by-side next to a straightened colon and the spine, we can see direct correlations between every part of our body in each structure. In other words, the eye at three o'clock may show weakened or inflamed tissue in the lung area while the transverse colon shows toxicity in the same area and the spine reflects pain or misalignment at T3. When we put these three puzzle pieces together and ask the right questions, we begin to map the cause of a problem, and can directly change the course of the dis-ease. If we remove the lung or part of the colon, the iris shows the loss as not only scar tissue, but also an absence of connective energy. We break the network that makes us whole, and the eye may be the only reminder or proof.

Cataracts, of course, can cloud the entire iris, and can be a strong indicator of many years of dehydration or toxicity. This is also important to understand when we look at the health of our pets or other animals. Dogs that develop cataracts are not just "growing old," but are exhibiting the results of many years of toxic food, air and/or water that have affected their entire body.

Like foot reflexology, chiropractic, energy modalities, massage and other body therapies, iridology needs to be understood as the gift it is. We are able to heal ourselves if we know what to look for and begin to change our habits and lifestyles before irreparable damage is done.

CHAPTER IV

No book on holistic or alternative health should be written without devoting a considerable amount of thought to water. Earth is approximately 80% water, most of it salt water, and our lives revolve around this fascinating compound. We grow into human beings while immersed in water, and the Earth allows us to continue life through the hydrological patterns of water recycling. We thirst for it, swim in it, bathe in it, build our houses close to it and sometimes suffer from its power. Our bodies depend on it, and we take it for granted.

It is the universal solvent and its molecular structure makes it totally unique. It is the most important key to life. Water is in the streams and rivers, under the ground, in the clouds, and frozen into the polar geography.

We watch the weather to be sure we can travel or tan, and get depressed if it rains too long. Some shudder at thunderstorms, and winter storms make us shiver. Water is the best conductor of electricity and can help to heighten our awareness and our connection to Heaven.

Native Americans revered water, and many tribes attributed names to its various forms. Water was the highest of all the elements, capable of changing its form and shape. The Greeks had Thor and Zeus, as the power of water and weather was held in high esteem. We build bridges over water, bottle it, carry it, dam it, channel it, fish in it, sail it, float in it – but somehow over time, we have lost respect for it.

We've replaced it with sodas and alcohol, allowed factories to dump anything and everything into it, watched as children of any age relieved themselves in it, wondered how nuclear waste polluted it. Because we're so technologically intelligent, we have found ways to pollute it even more with hormonal waste, antibiotics, and antidepressants, chemicals most have never heard of, and even the agents that are supposed to protect us from disease.

There are more than 700 chemicals in the water supplies that feed our homes and businesses, most of which have been proven to be carcinogenic, or at the least, dangerous to our health. Heavy toxic metals such as mercury and lead are released through mining. The Pecos River in New Mexico was once a pristine source of water, but is now so contaminated from mining pollution that residents along its course cannot use well water or eat the fish that somehow survive in it.

Oil drillers had brine pits for runoff, and farmers added to the pollution with herbicides and pesticides. Deforestation has caused massive erosion of ground soil and the drainage systems that empty into rivers and streams are filled with lawn fertilizers, extraordinary amounts of animal waste, and other chemicals that flow like rivers back to the ground.

Landfills in New York State made the news in the 1970's and 80's when residents of Love Canal were forced to leave their homes, many leaving behind the gravesites of children. There are thousands of landfills all over the United States, and the leaching effect these chemicals and radioactive compounds have on the groundwater will continue for hundreds of years. Many believe this is another case of, "someone else's job." As long as we don't believe we're directly affected, we won't worry about it.

Another belief is that wastewater and treatment plants are there to make the water safe, so there's nothing to worry about. This is partially correct. Billions of gallons of chlorine, for example, are dumped into our drinking water to make it "safe" to drink. Chlorine was used in World War I to kill people, and it does kill the living organisms that are in the water at the plant. The problem is, chlorine also has lethal by-products and we ingest them, bathe in them, and release them into the air as toxic gases when we boil them.

Have you ever wondered why the cancer death rate has decreased while the cancer incident has tripled since 1960? Has it bothered you that heart and lung disease, arteriosclerosis, arthritis, colon and liver cancer, and a host of other diseases and illnesses are on the rise in spite of the thousands of new drugs introduced each decade? Did God intend birds to get the flu or cows to be diseased?

Every bit of the water on Earth is connected. Every weather system connects our toxic waste to each other. The Earth's natural recycler of evaporation and precipitation is universal, and the winds of change carry our mistakes in all directions.

Hurricanes, typhoons and tornadoes are the most violent storms and the United States is the only country that has tornadoes. These cyclones, cycles of change, are destructive and sometimes deadly, but what can we learn from them? We seem to believe that the Earth is separate from us, and that all the weather we endure or enjoy is not really connected to our bodies or minds. We each have our own hurricanes, our own tornadic changes that come from our imbalances in energy. As the Earth does what it needs to do to heal itself, so do our bodies, sometimes because we direct it, but more often because it's the body's job to do whatever it has to do to stay on Earth. The more we pollute the earth, the more tornadic the storms. The more we pollute ourselves, the more frequent and tornadic the dis-ease.

Our answer to polluted water has been a deluge of bottled water products that have made many companies very prosperous, but done nothing to keep us well. Some people say they boil their water and believe that to be safe, unaware that boiling toxic water in your home releases toxic gases into the air. Others buy distilled water because they're sure there's nothing harmful left from this process. This is mostly true. The harmful contaminants have been distilled, but the bottles are cleaned with chlorine, and the water itself contains none of the minerals we should have. It's essentially dead water.

Some people have learned to dislike the taste of water, most likely because the salt purifiers of the fifties and the chlorination from the sixties until now, has left them with this distaste. They use soda and tea and coffee and beer and wine to make up for the lack of water. Water is two parts hydrogen and one part oxygen. Anything that changes this chemically makes it something other than water. The biggest killer in the United States is not cancer or heart disease, but dehydration.

Coffee, the mainstay of morning rush hour, is a diuretic. It makes you eliminate even more water from your system. Our cells depend on water and minerals to function. If we are not replenishing our own water table with fresh, healthy water, how can we not know that the streams we call arteries and veins, and the ocean we call brain are not drying up and polluted? Coffee and caffeine also leach minerals from our bodies such as calcium and magnesium, essential to heart and muscle heath.

Because our skin is the largest organ of our body, we are constantly absorbing pollutants and chemicals in every shower and bath. We step into a hot shower, which opens the pores, and absorb within ten minutes the equivalent of three to four pounds of water laced with chlorine and a host of chemicals that no one even tests. We cover ourselves with creams and lotions hoping that the miracle of chemicals will hydrate and restore our skin to health. We have pieces of our colons surgically removed because dehydration has formed pockets of toxic waste when all we had to do was drink good water to keep it clean and healthy.

Every animal and plant on Earth depends on water to give it life. Organic farming is not the answer to healthy vegetables if the water tables are polluted. Bottled water is not the answer if the water is dead or dangerous chemicals have to be used to clean the containers. Carbon filters in refrigerators are not the answer as they not only need to be changed or cleaned often to avoid molds and bacteria, but they essentially only remove the chlorine and not other volatile organic compounds. Carbon filter pitchers and ceramic containers are not the answer either for many of the same reasons.

The Earth cleans our water through a very slow process of mineralization, ionization and electro-static filtering. Because the earth has many layers, water flows through it and into it slowly, taking its time to reach the aquifers. A quick pour through a carbon filter or crushed ice from the refrigerator is not going to provide safe, healthy water.

The best water system is one that mimics the Earth and has an automatic back-flushing capability to ensure clean media. A KDF carbon block filter is a good beginning. It uses an electrochemical oxidation process that destroys bacteria, volatile organic compounds, removes chlorine and its by-products, and reduces many other chemicals. It needs a second stage carbon filter of high quality to trap known and unknown germ spores and toxic molds. It needs enough time for the water to flow through it, which means it can't just be a showerhead or faucet attachment. The media need to be large enough to last a long time and to continuously clean water during emergency storm conditions when water is deemed unsafe.

Few companies can provide this system, but those that do should be considered Godsends. Don't be fooled by claims that carbon is everything and a small carbon filter will keep you healthy. There are hundreds of lawsuits pending against many companies who have made these claims, and many people have paid the price.

If you still believe your water is safe and healthy, or that water purifying is "someone else's job," at least get educated enough, and take suitable action, to protect your children and grandchildren. That IS your job.

Healthy water is a good start, but what do we do about food? The physical and mental body depends on food for essential nutrients, minerals and enzymes provided by the Earth and God. Because our water tables that feed our root systems and sprinkler systems are contaminated, our food is also becoming toxic and unable to hold nutrients as was intended. Pesticides and herbicides are abundantly used to control insect infestation and grow larger fruits and vegetables. Organic foods avoid chemicals, but are subject to water pollution and transportation contaminants. Unless you are using a whole-house water system to clean your water, and have avoided runoff in your own garden, homegrown vegetables, though the safest, are still prone to toxicity.

Special diets that call for more meat and fewer vegetables and fruits are even more hazardous, as animals feed on chemically treated food, waste products and toxic wastewater before being slaughtered and shipped to our tables.

Steaming or boiling vegetables to retain what we can of their nutrients means exposing us and our food to boiled chemical compounds that release toxic gases. It all gets a little depressing, doesn't it?

Case Study

Margaret T., age 56, came for a consultation in June 2000. She complained of leg cramps and pain, swollen knees, headaches and an overall feeling of "achiness." She had been to several doctors who tested her thyroid, performed an MRI and ran the regular scope of blood tests. Their findings were generally inconclusive, but they told her she was probably menopausal and should consider hormone therapy. Her legs were not only swollen, but also discolored in varying degrees.

The MRI showed some calcium deposits in the third and fourth cervical area, but was otherwise negative. Her doctors told her she had arthritis.

My questions included diet, water, supplementation and medications. She was no longer taking any vitamin supplements and had refused hormone therapy. She was adamant that her drinking water was pure. I asked about dental work. She insisted her teeth were in great shape as she had just completed a dental visit and everything checked out fine.

Her fingernails showed weakness in the small and large intestines, so I checked her eyes uses iridology. The right iris at 1.8 pointed to congestion and weakness in the lower jaw and the left iris showed the same at 10.7 for the upper jaw. I again asked about her teeth, and again she said she was convinced everything was fine. The lymphatic system indicators in her eyes showed a cloudiness that often points to a labored immune system and a possible systemic infection. She informed me her white blood count was slightly elevated.

After many more questions about possible injuries or past infections, I went back to the jaw areas and asked more specific questions about her teeth. She then informed me that she had several crowns. When I checked for the placement of the crowns, they were in the same areas that showed weakness in her eyes. I suggested she return to her dentist to have the teeth checked under the crowns. I also suggested that others who had possible systemic infections, especially from dental problems, had positive results from using Golden Seal Root in capsule form for 5-7 days. My last suggestion was to check her drinking water. She once again said her drinking water was fine as it was city tap water and they said it was safe.

Ten days later, she called to inform me of her progress. She had returned to her dentist who once again told her the teeth and crowns were perfect. Trusting herself more than his statements, she received a second opinion from an orthodontic surgeon who discovered minute, but decisive cracks beneath the crowns of two teeth. One tooth was in the lower right jaw, the other in the upper left. He repaired the teeth and replaced the crowns.

She decided to try Golden Seal to cleanse her blood and took two capsules for five days. She also decided to try bottled water instead of tap water to see if it made a difference.

Three months later, she called again to tell me she felt great, her edema was gone and the discoloration had finally gone away. She had suffered with her symptoms for more than a year and visited four doctors, two clinics and a psychiatrist.

The better model for this particular case would have been a full check-up from a physician to alleviate any concern for acute or life threatening conditions. A referral to a holistic consultant for a full history and alternative indicators would have aided the physician in possibly referring to a dentist, or drawing more conclusions from x-rays of the upper and lower jaw and treating accordingly.

My time with Margaret was less than two hours for the initial consultation. Follow-up consisted of three 10-15 minute "check-ups." She receives regular massage therapy and maintains her health with vitamin supplementation, healthy water and exercise.

Though we need to take action on the condition of our water and the Earth, there's no reason for depression. God knew we were going to do all the things we've done and so created us with physical layers and back-up systems, creative energies, and in many of us, strong constitutions. We will find the way if we remain open to the answers. We'll be led in the right direction if we trust and believe. But we have to keep our eyes on the keys. Taking extra Vitamin C is not going to protect you from chemical toxicity if your body doesn't have time to cleanse. Cleansing diets are not going to protect you if you refill with toxic water. Nothing is going to make you feel better or help you to heal if you don't believe in what you're doing or that you will be well.

Vitamin and herbal supplements gained increased

popularity in the early eighties as health food franchises and leftover vegetarians from the sixties demanded alternatives to traditional health care. Even in the fifties, we heard about iron supplements for anemia and the multiple vitamin that was all we needed for longevity. Food companies jumped on the bandwagon with advertisements for breads and cereals that promised to supply the essential twelve vitamins and minerals. Water softeners were abundant as the clothes industry flourished and people clamored for sudsier water for less money. The softeners added salt to the water and swollen ankles, bloated bellies, and a thirst for anything but water became the norm. Soda was the chosen drink for decades with no thought of the damage from sugar or carbonation. A few households still insisted on cod liver oil as a daily supplement to promote strong bones, especially after the polio scare that produced a President in a wheelchair.

Vitamins are food. Minerals are part of the food and essential for vitamin absorption and efficiency. Herbs are medicine. So many take a combination of herbs and vitamins on a daily basis, not realizing that they are essentially "dosing" with medicine in an attempt to alleviate symptoms. Allopathic medicine does the same thing, substituting natural ingredients from plants with laboratory, synthetic copycats that do not contain the original properties of the plants. What kind of vitamins should you be taking and which ones?

Vitamins need to come from natural sources, not the laboratory. God put many extra catalysts in fruits and vegetables to make sure we absorbed them and they performed the way they should perform. Laboratories only use the basic chemical compound and ignore the God-given extras. Natural vitamins are more expensive, but how much are you worth? Liquid vitamins are the most readily absorbed, but beware of chlorine or other harmful products that have been added for who knows what reason. One shot glass full of liquid vitamins a day is all a healthy person needs to stay that way. For those of you who have bottles stacked in your cupboard, start over.

When we are basically healthy, drinking water, getting exercise and are aligned, we only need a good vitamin/mineral supplement to keep us going and protect us. Of course, most people who have finally turned to alternative medicine are already in a deteriorated physical and mental state and may need a few extra supplements to get them back on track.

Knowing which extra vitamins to take is not always an easy task. Pharmaceutical companies that now produce almost as many vitamins as they do drugs, rely on the average person to be uneducated and confused about supplements. You'll buy more and buy often if you keep the symptom-cure headset. All they have to do is get you fearful about your future to ensure a sale. Someone tells you about an article touting vitamin C as a cure-all for colds or stress, and you buy the garden variety at the local grocery store and take a few dozen a day for protection.

Herbs are a little more dangerous. Herbs are medicine and no one, despite the present mindset, should be on any medication very long. Vitamin compounds laced with herbs like Echinacea or ginseng can cause a host of problems in people who already have weaknesses in the circulatory or immune systems. These herbs are temporary medicines that should be used a maximum of 10 to twenty days, yet millions of Americans ingest them with their multiple vitamins every day. Very few people have ever died from herbs as discontinuing them removes the side effects almost immediately. They're not drugs. But many people will find themselves searching for new herbs or miracle cures with each new symptom and lose hope that herbal remedies may provide relief.

Every vitamin needs some other vitamins and minerals to work effectively in our bodies. Even scientists used to know this, as they were the ones who extracted the compounds from the plants and reproduced them in labs. They knew spinach contained Vitamin A and Iron, and we learned from Popeye that spinach would make us strong. I remember learning to love spinach because of that cartoon. What we didn't know was that spinach won't work by itself. Vitamin A needs the C, D, and E vitamins along with calcium, magnesium, and manganese to be properly absorbed and utilized. Iron needs selenium, and then the C, D, and E vitamins need other minerals and vitamins. A multiple, synergistic compound is the best answer to balancing these supplements.

Many people believe they don't need supplements because they eat a balanced diet and get all of the nutrients they need. Think again. Vegetables and fruits still rely on our water table, and because of pollution and contaminants, that water table no longer provides the nutrients we need to survive. Add the herbicides and pesticides to our dinner table and we end up needing more healthy water to flush them out, and a supplement program to keep us alive.

Revelation 22:2 "The leaves of the tree are for the healing of the nations." Christians have known about and heard of the essential oils that come from plants since the beginning of Christianity, but it was the Creator, God, who made the plants that surround us and gave us everything we need to heal and be healed. The oils from the plants are aromatic, but more importantly, they are the blood of the plant and contain the unique energetic, vibrational properties that only God could create. The frequencies of essential oils are higher than the frequency in most of the organs in our bodies, only of course, if the oils are obtained correctly and not synthetic or manmade.

When we venture into a garden and smell a rose, we awaken a part of our brain that resonates to the aroma, is in harmony with the vibration. The scent can carry us to memories of love or dreams of paradise. A rose can remind us of a funeral or a wedding or a special date, but those are aromatic memories. The therapeutic properties are much different and have no connection to memory.

Ancient Egyptians used frankincense in their halls of worship to uplift their spirits and enable a meditative state. Frankincense was given to Jesus, according to Christians, and many feet of ancient Babylon, Israel and Rome were anointed with oils. Indeed, the Garden of Eden was our intended dwelling, devoid of roads and cars and pollution, filled with plants and trees and flowers imbued with the powers of God to heal us or keep us well. Since we are energy and need to maintain a specific range of frequencies to be considered "alive," the vibrations and properties of plants, fruits and vegetables are essential to our existence.

By the way, children's vitamins are absolutely dangerous because of the sugar content and dosage amounts. They're not balanced and probably have as much nutritional value as a bite of an apple and a small carrot. Children are not ruling adults. They will learn at an early age that fruits and vegetables taste good, that water is really necessary and quenches your thirst, that candy may be a once or twice-a-year treat, and that vitamin supplements may not look or taste like candy at all.

My older brother wasn't allowed to drink carbonated beverages and had very little candy as a child. He's almost sixty at the time of this writing and still has no cavities.

My grandfather had water and an apple every morning, walked to work, and made sure he had vegetables every night. He lived to be well over a hundred years old.

We take better care of our cars, lawns and dogs than we do of our children. We would never carbonate and sugar the grass, or feed candy to the dog. If a warning light flashes on the SUV dashboard, we make special time to take it in for service, but when our children flash warnings and begin to break down, we fill them up with whatever is convenient and fast, tell the day care people or teachers to make sure they get their medication, and then tell them we love them by taking them out for ice cream. Somewhere between the fifties and the new millennium, we switched from spinach to sugary, synthetic characters. Maybe we should look a little harder at our own evolution.

Food is energy. It has a vibration, a frequency, and a color. Each chakra needs specific foods to feed and complement it. Green foods, like broccoli, peas, beans, and kale give us the necessary vibration to feed the heart, lungs and upper thoracic vertebrae of the spine. These vegetables also contain the harmonic of yellow and feed the solar plexus area and the related organs. Red foods are not as abundant, but also serve their purpose in the digestive areas and the complementary cervicals. Red, orange, yellow, green, blue, purple and white. If we eat a balance of color, we have a balanced diet that enables all of our energy centers to work at peak efficiency.

Television came to America in nineteen forty-nine, and with it came T.V. dinners, splintered family time, potpies and the beginning of the obesity movement. Prior to this, children often had part-time jobs or chores to be done after school. When they weren't working, they were playing, as children should. Not video games or online trivia, but the games that stretched their bodies, increased their circulation, strengthened the heart and pushed oxygen to the brain.

The sixties and seventies saw the women's movement get Mom out of the kitchen and into the work force. Latchkey kids began fending for themselves and the easiest food for them to prepare was peanut butter sandwiches and ice cream. Fast food restaurants sprang up all over the country and touted timesaving meals on the run, meals full of carbohydrates and fats, as they were also the easiest to prepare. Fruits and vegetables became things only grandma ate, and fried chicken, burgers and fries became the mainstay of children's diets.

Schools also changed. Many stopped serving hot lunches and opted instead for delivered pizza and stale sandwiches. Lunch bags were easier to fill with Twinkies™ and candy, and because kids were reacting to the loss of parental guidance and supervision, toys and more candy were added to the bags as appeasement. The women's movement was a good thing in many ways, but men didn't pick up the slack. Their days for babysitting were weekends, and televised sports became their recreation, along with popcorn, pizza and soda for refreshment, readily shared with any children who may interrupt a game.

Juvenile diabetes was on the increase, as were heart attacks, cardiovascular disease, colon cancer and high blood pressure. We didn't listen. Because we didn't know how or didn't want to deal with our guilt, we kept providing more treats and hoped that somehow our kids would still love us. Our frequency was greatly diminished, and because of too many sugars and carbohydrates, full of static. We gave this energy to our children, at birth, and every day since they joined us as humans. ADD became an accepted classification for more and more children. Listen to the words: Attention Deficit Disorder. Whose attention was missing? Instead of giving them the attention that we as adults seek from guides, teachers, and our highest parent, we gave them medication to calm them down.

Being someone's child is the one thing the entire human race has in common. If we believe in God, the Creator, we relate to Him as Father. And to those who believe in Mary, we often call her Mother. We are unconditionally loved by a higher power. As parents, we also love our children unconditionally. We know they will somehow break some rules and will invariably get into trouble. We know they'll test some of the basic commandants, and we should know they expect us to react. We don't want them to lie, yet we lie to them. We don't want them to steal, but they watch us applaud the actors in movies or on television who do steal and get away with it. We want them to respect us, but we continually disrespect each other be it spouse, friend, employer or stranger. Thou shalt not kill, unless we condone it and pay to watch it.

It could be so easy. How hard is it to not break a promise or not even make a promise if you don't know you can keep it? How hard is it to be truthful, first with yourself, then with others? Why is it okay for so many to ignore their mother or swear at their father when these are the ones who co-created us and gave us life? Why do we pray to be heard, and then fail to listen even to each other?

Case Study

David C., age 38, complained of rectal bleeding, an overactive libido, abdominal pain, recurring respiratory infections and occasional dizziness. Repeated visits to clinics and hospitals and several colonoscopy exams revealed the possibility of Crohn's disease, but gave no indicators for the other symptoms. David tried chelation therapy, which only alleviated some of the symptoms for a short time. He also tried massage therapy, Rolfing, and trigger-point therapy, again with limited results.

My initial interview lasted a little more than three hours, as David was unable to clearly recall many things from the past. Iridology showed a spastic, distended and sluggish colon, especially in the ascending colon area. 6.0 on the left iris showed an almost silver luminescence, something I had not seen before.

Kinesiology was used to test for metal toxicity and indicated possible silver, lead and nickel toxicity. Upon this finding, I reverted to more history. David suddenly remembered that he had contracted malaria during military service and also had an ankle injury with a pin insertion. That explained the silvery hue at 6.0.

There appeared to be minimal absorption of vitamins and minerals evidenced by his finger and toenails, and his hair. Water consumption was minimal. David drank "a lot" of iced tea as he also worked outside in Alabama and believed tea was a good substitute for water. When further discussing his work we discovered that he often worked with pesticides in his greenhouse; however, his bouts with pneumonia did not seem to coincide with the pesticide usage.

Additional iridology and kinesiology revealed probable Candida and parasite invasion in the intestines, liver, gall bladder and lung/bronchial area.

Palpation and massage revealed high-density congestion in the entire abdominal region and slight discoloration on the left ankle. Massage also revealed spinal misalignment in the T-3 through T-8 regions and L5-S1.

His physicians had recommended colon surgery to remove "deteriorated portions of the colon" and a possible colostomy to alleviate the bleeding. David chose to find alternatives so, in lieu of surgery, they recommended Maalox and avoidance of alcohol and coffee.

The first course of action was to alleviate the colon's acute condition to enable any further herbal or mineral supplementation to be absorbed. We decided to try six ounces of George's aloe vera juice 3 times a day to reduce the inflammation, along with liquid acidophilus to replace the intestinal flora and protect him from infection. Immediate referral to a chiropractor was recommended for the spinal misalignment. We also decided his diet needed extensive changes. We decided on a sugar-free, dairy-free diet and the elimination of acid producing food or drink i.e. coffee, tea, soda, alcohol, tomatoes, corn. Lemon water was suggested to reduce mucous and deter the possibility of kidney/gall stones. He was told to return in one week.

After seven days, iridology confirmed that the initial two chiropractic adjustments had begun to realign the spine. Rectal bleeding had slowed to a once every three days rate. We decided on another week of the same therapy with the addition of a liquid vitamin/mineral to further protect him from infection.

After ten more days, he was able to change his chiropractic appointments to twice a month as his spine was holding the adjustments well. The chiropractor agreed that he needed additional counseling on nutrition and herbal therapies along with massage or other bodywork to help restore abdominal tone.

After thirty days, David was no longer bleeding and his abdominal pain was minimal, though he complained of occasional intensified pain in the upper right abdominal quadrant. We added an herbal colon conditioner for 30 days to prepare his colon for cleansing and also began a parasite cleanse at a suggested ten day on, ten day off regimen. All previous suggestions were maintained.

Palpation of the upper right abdominal quadrant revealed the possibility of gall stone formation. Iridology confirmed an inherent weakness in the gallbladder area. We added a ten-day gallbladder therapy consisting of drinking two parts olive oil to one part lemon juice before morning food and the last thing before retiring.

He returned in 24 days and stated he felt better than he had in seven years. Further testing showed Candida and parasites were reduced, but not gone, the gall bladder area was no longer congested or inflamed, bowel movements had become more regular without bleeding, and the abdomen was less distended.

We began an intensified colon cleanse, restarted the parasite cleanse and referred back to the chiropractor to maintain spinal integrity. Gall bladder therapy was discontinued, vitamins/minerals were maintained as were the acidophilus and aloe vera.

In twenty-one days, David returned and said he had seen "white things" in his fecal matter, which may have indicated expelled parasites, but he now felt great.

His only maintenance is now a twice a year chiropractic visit, regular massage/reflexology sessions, vitamin/mineral therapy, a more balanced diet and additional "as needed" therapies after pesticide usage. We also recommended, by the way, that he either change his line of work, or find an alternative to pesticides.

His chiropractor was completely cooperative and agreeable to a complementary therapy approach to his problems. His physicians, however, were not happy with his choices. Though he now tested "healthy," and wanted to share what he had learned with his medical doctors, they refused to listen and left him with free samples of antacids because his problems would "probably return."

Case Study

Susan G., age 74, complained of dizziness, alternating constipation/diarrhea and pneumonia whenever she traveled to visit her grandchildren in Texas. Several physicians had recommended a colonoscopy, which she refused. She had been on antibiotic therapy four times in the past 16 months for pneumonia. She was not a smoker or in any high-risk group for upper respiratory ailments. Her legs and hands had small red and black streaks and discoloration in different areas.

Both the left and right iris showed a spastic colon with considerable sluggishness and debris. They also showed several pockets that had parasitic indicators. Her fingernails revealed non-absorption of minerals and her lymphatic and circulatory systems showed up cloudy with iridology.

After an extensive history, I concentrated on her drinking water. She assured me her water was "the best." I asked what water she drank when she went to Texas and she said tap water and it was "good." I went back to her local drinking water and discovered she was drinking tap water at home also.

Using kinesiology, I tested her for parasites and her body indicated positive. I then asked if she had any animals at home or ever went barefoot. She said, "No." Together we asked her body about her drinking water and the indicator was negative, in this case indicating an aversion to her present drinking water. We then asked about Texas drinking water and received the same indication.

She had spent several thousand dollars and traveled to a few famous clinics to resolve this problem. Together we decided to attack the water situation and to rid the body of any parasites that may have invaded.

We purchased three gallons of spring water, a tincture of black walnut and wormwood, a quart of George's aloe vera juice and a good liquid vitamin with minerals. She took the black walnut-wormwood tincture every 3 hours for three days and consumed only spring water. She took 4 oz. of aloe vera in the morning and evening to soothe the bowel and on the third day started her liquid vitamins.

Within seven days, all the discoloration in her legs had disappeared and her bowel habits had started to normalize. We added olive leaf extract and cloves to destroy any remaining parasites, and increased the spring water ingestion to two gallons a day.

Ten days later a check of her eyes showed most of the cloudiness clear in her lymphatic and circulatory systems and she felt generally better. We stopped the black walnut-wormwood tincture and began ingestion of liquid acidophilus to replace the intestinal flora. We also did a Candida cleanse as the repeated antibiotic therapy had caused a massive yeast condition.

She doesn't come for therapy very often now because she has eleven grandchildren in Texas and she's always there. Her postcards indicate she's drinking water that is "really good," and she feels great.

It should seem pretty clear that a simple solution to many of our health problems would be to begin with making sure we're drinking and bathing in healthy water. If we're 80% water, this simple step could take care of a large percentage of our problems. Another fairly simple answer could be the elimination of ego, especially when it comes to our bodies and our health. Complementary, alternative medicine, which incorporates truly holistic therapies, could save consumers millions of dollars, reduce the costs of health insurance, save many lives, and restore some faith in western medicine.

CHAPTER V

Now it's time to begin your earth walk. As we have said, we are all a part of this earth we walk on, created with love, and intended to live abundantly and with joy. Every tree, every blade of grass, every ocean, river, stream, animal, and cloud is a part of us. To understand ourselves and learn how to not only heal, but to stay well, we have to feel our connection to the earth, and to Heaven.

Every tree has a meaning. Every flower has an essence that resonates. Every plant or weed is filled with lifeblood similar to ours, and all of these things were created for a reason. Not one thing in our lives is a mistake. Nothing is useless. Remember that when you look in the mirror. The reflection you see is just that, a reflection of all that is. Our chakra energies are the mirror reflections of rainbows and every vibration a reflection of God or the Universe. Call the higher power that gave you life whatever you like and don't worry about the sex or gender. These are earthly worries, created for the continuance of life. God's gender is universal.

We, too, have both male and female energies, and in the

first nine weeks after conception have no defined gender. It is only when our soul receives its purpose that we become either female or male, and our path is created with all the obstacles, lessons, realities and truths belonging to that energy. As we grow and unfold in the womb, we're like flowers with both male and female characteristics. At a chosen time, one energy supercedes the other because our future and the generations after us will depend on the reproduction of those energies.

Think of it this way. Everything on Earth strives for balance. Night becomes day, darkness becomes light, fear and love are emotions, or energy in motion, predators become prey, children become parents, and the cycle continues. Male energy needs female energy and vice versa. Not external sources of energy, but internal. Every boy has an inner girl. Every woman has an inner man.

Some men in our world appear or act more feminine. Their external or expressive energies are considered more female in nature. They're nurturing, giving, gentle. Some judge these men and say they're not man enough. Those who understand God know that the male energy inside must be balanced by the external energy, and therefore, they are truly male.

Some women appear "sexy" and outrageously beautiful. Inside, many are the "doers" or the "fixers," possessing the male energy that makes them admired mothers, respected leaders. The female energy must be balanced.

We strive for this balance in relationship to each other. We search for our soul mate, believing this to be one and only one ever created just for us. We long for a relationship with our other half, someone to complete us, make us whole. This is our first lesson. We need a relationship to ourselves, a completion, an understanding and an unconditional love of the reflection in the mirror, before we can ever secure a relationship with anyone or anything else on earth. Only when we are secure with our reflection, our true being, can we love completely. The person looking back at you is your best friend, your advisor, and your confidant. That being you're looking at was with you at birth and is always with you. You are your own child and a child of God.

Begin your earthwalk by loving yourself, not with ego or false pride or bravado, but with unconditional truth. If you are afraid, face your fear. If you feel shame or anger or hatred for yourself, know that these emotions also come from fear and face them. If you don't believe you deserve to be loved, or that you're "good" enough, or that you're as beautiful, handsome, or smart as someone else, face these feelings and know that they, too, come from fear and not love.

Look that reflection in the eye and say, "I love you. I will never hurt you, or deny you, lie to you, steal from you or kill you. You are my best friend and I'll do everything I can to keep you well and happy and full of joy."

Look harder and say, "I forgive you."

The mind, the body, and the spirit need to hear you and feel you loving yourself before they can work with you to help you heal and keep you well. Look in the mirror every single day and let that special person know how important and necessary and wonderful they are.

Once we've taken a good look at ourselves, we need to better understand our relationship to nature. Despite or because of the weather, go outside. A part of you is every tree, every flower, and every animal. Native Americans respect the spirit in every living thing and teach us to honor the gifts from the Creator.

Maple trees show us that change can be beautiful, and that life, as we know it may end, but spring always brings rebirth. The armadillo sleeps on its back exposing its soft underbelly. He teaches us that vulnerability is a part of life and may help us to learn trust and faith. The hawk has keen vision and sees all things while also picking out details. Looking at the whole picture can teach us to heal. Rose bushes have thorns, but we give the flowers to represent our love, reminding us that love should have no conditions. The rose also teaches us strength through silence. The word silent is an anagram for listen, and only when we are truly silent, can we hear the messages from Mother Earth.

Daffodils push through the snow announcing preparedness for spring. Their yellow horns teach us to face each new day with courage. All trees have roots and proudly reach toward Heaven, swaying in the wind and branching in all directions. Evergreens teach us balance between our emotions and physical pain. They withstand the winter and the changes of the seasons without losing their presence or their color. Aspen trees teach us about our connection to each other. Though each individual tree is unique, each is connected to all other aspens through their root systems.

Many animals teach us the basic rules, and God smiles a little when we finally catch on. If you steal, a raccoon will be your totem, as he is the masked robber who scurries in the night. If you put too much energy into storing and saving your worldly goods, you are like the squirrel and will someday learn that you no longer remember where you've hidden your wealth.

Even weeds have lessons. Dandelions populate our yards in the spring, and we hasten to kill them with chemicals. Dandelion roots are blood cleansers, given to us to clean our bloodstreams after the long winter. Milk thistle, another weed, cleanses the liver, and peppermint can soothe the stomach and intestines.

What do you see when you look around you? If you have a dog by your side, you are being given loyalty and unconditional love. If the sky is blue, it's reflecting the oceans and seas that surround us, and is also a reflection of the water within us, our communication through the power of water. If a deer stands in front of you, she's reminding you to be gentle, with yourself and with others.

When you stretch your arms and reach for the sky, you are doing what every creature does every day. Stretching is one of the keys you need to heal. Your dog or cat stretches before sleeping, and as soon as they awake. Your bird stretches its wings, and even a whale will roll and stretch its flippers. Most people have gotten more aware of the need for exercise, but have forgotten entirely about stretching. Our joints, muscles, bones and circulatory system need to be stretched so that energy can flow unimpeded and the lymphatic system can continue cleansing.

Face the East as you stretch and give thanks for your breath. The East is the direction of new birth and sunshine, the home of the Eagle and the color orange. The East reminds us that all things come to a new day, and to be grateful for the first breath you take in the morning. Breathe deeply to expand your chest and lungs. Feel the energy of the air around you and within you. When we're depressed, tired, frustrated or afraid, the East lets us see the light. All things are cyclical and our circular path will always bring us back to this point. Don't be afraid of your pain or dis-ease. Breathe in all that the earth and God, the Creator, have given you. Fly high like the Eagle and soar above the feelings of abandonment or low self-esteem. Each day is the morning of the rest of your life. Instead of harboring negativity, let the sun rise and recharge you, even if it's behind a cloud or busy with a rainstorm. Even then the sun is still there.

Turn toward the South, and as you do, feel your connection to the Earth and its fire. You are a warm-blooded being and your body should reflect that warmth in every part of you. If your feet are cold, ask yourself first if you are afraid to move forward. If you have no fear, let the warmth from your heart fill your next step. You are on Earth for a reason, and part of every human's mission is to be a part of humanity. Earth is your partner and will help you.

The South is our soul, the color red. When we face the South, we ask the questions that have no answers, because the questions are the answers. Why are we here? Why do I hurt? When will I feel better? What's my purpose? Expect no response. By asking the questions, you are fulfilling one of the goals of our spirit. It is in the asking that we become who we were intended to be. The animal of the South is the coyote, the trickster. Don't let your mind interfere. This is not the direction for the mind. The mind will analyze and ask more questions that truly have no answers. The mind will trick you into believing you know more than the next person, more than your parents, more than your Creator. There is no room for control. Control is an illusion and is only possible if others allow it. Trusting the soul and its purpose is our sole reason for being. Trust your existence. Trust your intuition and experience. Don't think it. Feel it.

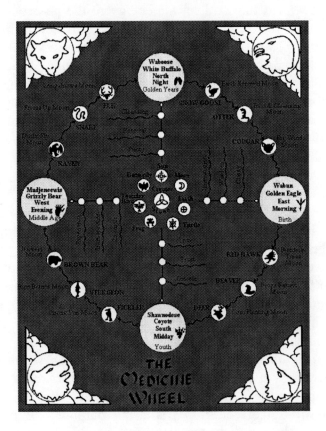

When you are comfortable in the presence of your spirit, turn toward the West. The bear retires to its cave, and so must you. Be still with yourself and listen to your body. Go into the darkness of the past. Don't be afraid. Things happened to you as a child. Memories of judgment, physical pain, fear, and loneliness. Your mother didn't hug you enough. Your father was too strict, or was never home. Your sister seemed more loved, or your brother was the favorite. Someone left you when you didn't think they should have. You tried to change someone, believing this was your mission and within your power. When they didn't change, or you couldn't save them, rescue them, mold them into your vision, your expectations broke your heart. You were always the one who had to care for everyone else. You carried the load, and it broke your back. You never felt support for anything you did, and now you carry the pain in your legs and your shoulders. You went to church, prayed for help and forgiveness, cried yourself to sleep and felt abandoned by God, and now your feet are swollen, your stomach is on fire and you're sure no one cares. All of these emotions and events have brought you to this moment, every moment a gift on your journey. Though some were painful, they were part of your process, your development, your reason. Take the lessons, and let go of the memory. If there are tears, let them be. If there is anger, let it be. If there is an overwhelming feeling of hopelessness or loss or unjust pain, let it be. Know that the cave is your sacred space, and as you go through the memories, you come closer to emerging from the darkness.

When you feel ready, turn toward the North, the healing direction, the home of the white buffalo, where night turns into day. Feel the strength that comes from knowing your beginning, your reason and your past. Let that energy flow through you and once again remind you that you are precious and unique and more than worth it. Clear your mind and your memory so only life can fill the void. Give your inner child the chance to make his or herself known. Our inner child allows us the freedom to play, to be truthful, and to look at life with a positive immortality. Nothing can harm us. There's no such thing as death or dying. This is the part of us that wants to live forever, and believes we can. This is also the part of us that cries out for attention, feels lost and confused, and needs a gentle hand.

So often we find ourselves tearful for no reason, or rebelling when we know we really don't want to. We get stubborn, jealous, envious, stomp our feet and "take the ball and go home." Our wounded inner child is always there and needs to be recognized. It is from this early energy that we begin the patterns of illness and disease.

Mom got scared when we fell, so every time we fall as adults, we also get scared. The other kids didn't want to play with us, so as adults we feel insecure in groups and shy at parties. We were laughed at when a pimple appeared on our cheek, so we spend thousands of hours in our lifetimes trying to cover every blemish, be it physical or emotional. Dad didn't like us to cry, or Grandma said, "be tough," so we armor ourselves and never show our emotions, even though emotions are the mainstay of our conscious energy.

Because no one ever asked us how we feel, we don't know. Because medicine was the answer to all our problems, we maintain our reliance on drugs. Because the uniforms of those in authority were drummed into our minds, we bow and obey to all white coats, black robes or prescription lettering.

Depression is your inner child being manipulative. Things haven't gone your way, or so you believe. You had expectations that life would be different, easier, more like someone else's, and life has let you down.

Listen. Be silent and listen to the love in your soul. Your life is exactly what it is supposed to be. We have choices. Most people believe free will is the choice to do whatever you want, and if it doesn't turn out the way you wanted it to, you believe you have the choice to manipulate a different ending. Sorry. Acting out your wants and desires with manipulation as the intention is not a choice. Acting them out in fear, with anger, with deception or malice is not a choice. Yes, we have the ability to create our lives, and re-create our paths, but if the intention is to change the will of God or our higher self, you will be defeated. Free will is only the choice between good and evil, and that becomes the choice between fear and love.

If God is love, and you choose any energy other than love-of self, of others, of life and of God- your choices will lead you to illness in your body, mind, and spirit. Time to grow up. That doesn't mean forget your youth, your younger self, that beautiful child within, but banish the brat, the bully, the manipulator, the liar and the cheat. Send those parts of you to a different plane, a different playground.

The possum plays dead to survive. If we play dead, we will surely die. The rat steals in the night and the weasel's slyness allows him to cheat his prey. Choose higher. Though all creatures are revered as teachers, choose to mimic those with strength, honor, fortitude, wisdom and courage.

We were born with faith and unconditional love. We were taught judgment, anger, fear, hatred, and distrust. As you begin your healing journey, go back and take the hand of your inner child. Ride the wind, lie in the grass, cloud walk, dance in the rain and smile at every new day.

This is the beginning of your Earthwalk. This is the road to the cause

CHAPTER VI

There are seven basic keys to finding the cause of illness or staying well. Seven is a sacred number, and to many, a lucky number. The keys are simple. Start with number one.

Water. The colon, brain, the entire body needs water. Not fluoridated, chlorinated water. Not water filled with disinfectant by-products or industrial waste. Clean, healthy water containing the minerals that make up the earth and our bodies. How do you get it and how much?

First of all, let's be clear on the amount of water the body needs. Holistically, every body is different, and every life is different, so the amount of water an individual needs will vary. The basic rule: Take half your body weight in ounces per day. If you weigh 150 pounds, you need seventy-five ounces of water per day. This will work if you are doing basic exercise, not living in extreme climates, not eating salty foods, don't have salt conditioners on your water supply, are not on medications, are not eating overly acidic foods, are not under extraordinary stress and are basically in balance. If you are not in balance, your water intake should increase gradually as you begin your earth walk

Bottled water will suffice until you can get a whole house

water system, but instead of storing your water in the big, plastic gallons or containers, transfer it to glass. The chlorine used to disinfect the plastic containers will leach into the water, and the by-products of chlorine will eventually kill you. Also, be sure to drink the water and not save it for a hurricane or a rainy day. The disinfectants will eventually dissipate, and stored water can contain harmful bacteria.

Drink your first glass of water as soon as you've stretched in the morning. Forget the coffee for a while. Coffee pulls calcium from the body and acts as a diuretic. It pulls fluid from the joints and leeches minerals from the muscles. That tired, achy feeling you have in the morning could be from the coffee you had the day before. You've been taught to rely on coffee or other stimulants to wake you up and get you "going." Teach yourself (and that special person in the mirror) that you don't need coffee any more. When you're well, and in balance, an occasional cup will be a treat.

Bathing or showering presents another problem. You may have a filter or pitcher for your drinking water, and we discussed earlier that these devices don't work, but what about your shower or bathtub? You absorb more chemicals, including chlorine by-products, in twenty-four showers than you do by drinking eight, 8 ounce glasses of water per day for five years. Your body is absorbing seven hundred or more chemicals every time you shower. Some scientists believe these chemicals don't stay in your body, and therefore, can't be harmful. Tell me why we have patches to quit smoking, and patches for hormone therapy, if chemicals don't absorb through the skin and get into our systems. Try weighing yourself before and after a twenty minute bath to see how much water you've absorbed. Health food stores and other distributors sell staged filters for the shower and promise they're ridding the water of everything harmful. Think about the layers of the earth and the amount of time it takes for water to be filtered by these layers. Does a six-inch filter do the same thing? You'll clean some of the chlorine and sediment, and that's better than nothing, but start saving for a better system. Beware of softeners and water conditioners that use salt, as these devices add salt to your diet and will eventually corrode your plumbing and dry your skin.

God gave us a world full of salt water and a small percentage of fresh water. Stay away from salt unless you're looking for a refreshing swim. Even then we need to shower afterward to remove the salt. Our bodies use a sodium-potassium pump within our cells to generate movement and life, but we don't need extra salt to make them work. When we cry, our tears are salty. When we perspire, we excrete salt and acids. When we urinate, we let go of acids and the vibrational energy associated with fear.

If your refrigerator contains a filter for water and ice, change it or clean it every month. You'll be amazed at the amount of bacteria that builds up just from glasses or hands touching the spout or spigot. These are only loose carbon filters that improve the taste of water and shouldn't be confused with a safe, healthy water system.

Boiling water releases harmful gases into the air and distilled water is essentially "dead" water containing none of the nutrients or electrical energy we need. Beware of water in restaurants and crushed ice or ice cubes as they may contain the most polluted water and often sit for hours in bacteria – laden containers.

Without water, we become the arid desert. The greatest cause of death in America is dehydration. Dehydration destroys heart muscle, colon membranes and liver cells. Dehydration deteriorates our eyes and allows toxins to build in the kidneys and bladder. Without water, your spine will begin to compress until you have bone-on-bone conditions, bone spurs and disc herniations. The heart needs electrical impulses to continue beating, and water is the conductor. Water conducts the vibrations of our emotions and balances our glands. Carbonated drinks, sugary soothers and milky thirst quenchers do nothing but add thickness to our arteries and cells, cause imbalances in the pancreas and circulatory system, and add sludge to the colon and intestinal walls. Our ankles swell, colons distend and bellies bloat because we thirst for water.

We are water. God gave us blue sky, clouds, rainstorms and rainbows to remind us of this vital connection. We recycle the water within our bodies, and throughout our planet. Houseplants, gardens, dogs and cats all depend on water. If you pour soda, coffee or tea on your plants, they'll die. If you give your pet fruit smoothies or beer or mocha shakes, it will get sick and die. If you bathe your children in chlorine, let them swim in chlorinated pools, and quench their thirst with soda, they may not outlive you.

Our minds and our brains can't live without water. Dehydration could be a cause of Alzheimer's, or at least, a contributing factor. We can't focus or think clearly, and when we do, our thoughts are negative or dry. We begin to think only of ourselves because we lack the property of water that allows us to expand and extend our universe. We become immersed and self-centered like small whirlpools spinning toward the drain. If our minds are out of balance, so too are our bodies and spirits as the triangular power is diminished and the trinity of life undermined.

Our souls also suffer without water. Tears of joy disappear. Sadness turns to anger and frustration when we can't spill the salt from our hearts. The vibrations of our chakras slow down, and our energy centers dim without the conductivity of water. We become shallow and dry, blowing in the dust instead of creating the winds of change. Our eyes begin to dry and we can't see the details of the miracles around us. The fine line between joy and despair disappears until we grow numb and can no longer react with the emotions that make us human. We can't feel. We don't feel the heartache of another person's loss or automatically jump for joy at someone's success. We become dead batteries with the hope of recharging at the next meal or church service or ball game.

So great is our need and dependence on water that it is mentioned in every religious or spiritual text, including Genesis and Revelations of the Bible. Christians are baptized in water and we flow from our mother's womb after the water "breaks." It is the first key to health, the first of seven.

CHAPTER VII

The second key is food. God gave us a smorgasbord of complete, balanced, and complementary wonders to ingest, and from that, we've created biochemical junk. Earth's food is a balance between alkaline and acid foods, with far more emphasis on alkaline. Disease has a very hard time existing in alkaline conditions, yet we do everything possible to make our bodies acidic. Red meat, French fries, alcohol, processed sugars, processed fats, carbonated soda, smoking, and drugs are the basics of acidity. The body needs to have a balanced Ph to stay healthy. We are, surely, what we eat.

Consider the chart below when choosing your menu for the day. Food combining is not a complicated science, but rather the art of choice. Study the chart and you'll learn that our society is one of poor choices.

Most Alkaline	Alkaline	Lowest Alkaline	FOOD CATEGORY	Lowest Acid	Acid	Most Acid
Stevia	Maple Syrup, Rice Syrup	Raw Honey, Raw Sugar	SWEETENERS	Processed Honey, Molasses	White Sugar, Brown Sugar	NutraSweet, Equal, Aspartame, Sweet 'N Low
Lemons, Watermelon, Limes, Grapefruit, Mangoes, Papayas	Dates, Figs, Melons, Grapes, Papaya, Kiwi, Blueberries, Apples, Pears, Raisins	Oranges, Bananas, Cherries, Pineapple, Peaches, Avocados	FRUITS	Plums, Processed Fruit Juices	Sour Cherries, Rhubarb	Blackberries, Cranberries, Prunes
Asparagus, Onions, Vegetable Juices, Parsley, Raw Spinach, Broccoli, Garlic	Okra, Squash, Green Beans, Beets, Celery, Lettuce, Zucchini, Sweet Potato, Carob	Carrots, Tomatoes, Fresh Corn, Mushrooms, Cabbage, Peas, Potato Skins, Olives, Soybeans, Tofu	BEANS VEGETABLES LEGUMES	Cooked Spinach, Kidney Beans, String Beans, Cooked Garlic	Potatoes (without skins), Pinto Beans, Navy Beans, Lima Beans	Chocolate
	Almonds	Chestnuts	NUTS SEEDS	Pumpkin Seeds, Sunflower Seeds	Pecans, Cashews	Peanuts, Walnuts, Peanut Butter
Olive Oil	Flax Seed Oil	Canola Oil	OILS	Corn Oil	Processed sprays	
None	None	Amaranth, Millet, Wild Rice, Quinoa	GRAINS CEREALS	Sprouted Wheat Bread, Spelt, Brown Rice	White Rice, Corn, Buckwheat, Oats, Rye	Wheat, White Flour, Pastries, Pasta
None	None	None	MEATS	Venison, Cold Water Fish	Turkey, Chicken, Lamb	Beef, Pork, Shellfish
	Breast Milk	Soy Cheese, Soy Milk, Goat Milk, Goat Cheese, Whey	EGGS/ DAIRY	Eggs, Butter, Yogurt, Buttermilk, Cottage Cheese	Raw Milk	Cheese, Homogenized Milk, Ice Cream
Herb Teas, Lemon Water, Water	Green Tea	Ginger Tea	BEVERAGES	Tea, Tap Water	Coffee	Beer, Soft Drinks

A food's acid or alkaline-forming tendency in the body has nothing to do with the actual pH of the food itself. For example, lemons are very acidic; however, the products they produce after digestion and assimilation are very alkaline, so lemons are alkaline-forming in the body. Likewise, meat will test alkaline before digestion, but it leaves very acidic residue in the body, so meat is very acid-forming.

The key, of course, is balance. An occasional cup of coffee, glass of beer, or a steak is not going to kill you, but Americans are not "occasional" when it comes to a poor diet. Bacon, eggs, white toast, butter, coffee, and a little sugar or aspartame are about as acidic as food gets, and that's just breakfast. Lunch might be a hamburger with fries and a diet soft drink, something we regularly feed our children. Add a little chicken for dinner with rice and a beer, and we have created an acidic condition that can begin to destroy our cells, tissues, and organs.

The reason we live as long as we do is that the body has a natural defense against acids, which is storing the acid in fat so it isn't able to permeate the cells. But it can't do this forever. Eventually, as we age, the cellular walls begin to break down and the acid corrosion destroys the cell itself. The body panics and tries to proliferate more cells to replace the ones that were destroyed. This is a symptom, and the name for it is cancer.

Acid burns. It causes inflammation, which in turn causes mucus, a defense the body uses to "cool the flames." Head colds, sinusitis, chest congestion, and constipation are all conditions exacerbated by mucus. Mucus attracts bacteria, viruses, yeast, molds, parasites, and fungus. These are living organisms, which love a warm, moist environment. Since most foods contain all of these critters, it would be wise to develop an environment they won't thrive in. When the body is alkaline, it readily flushes acid waste, which in turn cleans out the mucus and inhibits harmful agents from "setting up house."

The digestive system has natural hydrochloric acid, and cells eagerly use acid for energy, but it's the toxic waste that ends up in our tissues and continues to build. Lactic acid is a by-product of muscle contraction, evidenced by those who exercise or lift weights. This acid can be painful if not flushed from the tissues, one of the benefits of massage, and a positive result of drinking water.

Food combining and timing is an important key to balanced health. The Ph is changed if we eat proteins with starch, acidic fruit with alkaline vegetables, and is adversely affected by drinking fluids with meals. If we have a glass of water with dinner, we dilute the digestive enzymes and the hydrochloric acid. This slows the digestive process and increases the acid waste from the food. Add beer, wine, soda, or coffee to this process and you have essentially created a toxic acid pool. Not only will the stomach suffer, but also the liver, gallbladder, pancreas, spleen and intestines. Drink your fluids at least thirty minutes before a meal, and wait an hour or so after you eat. Food has no need to be "washed down," if it's chewed correctly and your body is functioning as it should be.

Why do we crave certain foods and have aversions to others? Food cravings can be learned, genetic, biological, chemical or psychological. Food is energy. We may crave steak because Dad used to grill steak the only days he was home. We crave salt because our minerals are out of balance and the sodium-potassium pump that keeps our cells going may trigger a sodium need. Sugar is a learned craving most often associated with comfort or reward. Craving chocolate may be an indicator of a hormonal imbalance; hence the box of chocolates on Valentine's Day. Coffee craving is an addiction to caffeine, often based on a psychological need to "face the day."

Addiction to eating is connected to physical, emotional, and spiritual imbalances. We never feel full, yet we're always "overstuffed." The void we believe to be in our stomachs is more likely in our attitude and our soul. We can't or don't want to digest everything we hear or see. We don't like what we see in the mirror, but we love every food placed in front of us.

We're fearful that we haven't done enough, been good enough, to get to Heaven, so we snack and find excuses for not going deeper into ourselves and churning away the garbage. We're full of doctrine and tenets, belief systems that agitate our digestive systems, our entire being. We say grace at the dinner table, and then stuff our bodies with useless calories. What we're saying is, thanks for the food you provided, but I'd rather have sugar and carbohydrates, or eat one of your animals for dinner. We think we're bored with life, or we're frustrated because life isn't as perfect as someone said it should be, so we eat. Eating fills the space, takes the time, and eventually makes us unable to enjoy life, so now we have an excuse.

Not eating is based on many of the same emotions, but reversed. When our hearts and souls feel full, we no longer hunger. Falling in love and having it reciprocated will fill the void, until we fear again. We fear the loss, the possible rejection, and we eat. When the loss is assumed, the rejection manifested, we eat, and then vomit, or excrete all we've taken in, so there'll be no evidence that we're looking to fill ourselves with love.

We eat socially and according to the menu or our finances, rather than being sociable and creating our own menus. We eat because we've set up a specific time when we are supposed to eat, rather than eating when we're hungry. We eat alone instead of sharing the gratitude for the day. We eat too early, too late, and too much. One helping doesn't quite do it, and we use the excuse that it tastes so good we just have to have more. Ah, the sweetness of life and living. If we could only savor this flavor as well.

So what is the right answer to balanced eating? Watch your pets and your kids and learn. Dogs and cats will drink water in the morning, and then wait a short time before eating. Kids are thirsty as soon as they wake up. Drinking water gets the digestive juices flowing and helps to neutralize any excess acid. Also worth noting is the fact that we are usually thirsty when we think we're hungry.

After neutralizing the excess acids, we want to cleanse the body. It has been resting and the immune system has been working hard to fight off intruders. Fruit is the best meal for the morning, but not fruit mixed with other foods. Because most fruit contains the same percentage of water as we do, we digest it quickly. If it sits "on top of" other foods, it will ferment and possibly cause gas or stomach upset. Eat fruit and wait thirty minutes before adding grains.

Many people feel they need protein for breakfast so they won't feel hungry. Proteins take longer to digest so we often have a "full" feeling, but making your body work that hard in the morning can make you tired by midday. When we're tired, we crave caffeine, so we grab a soda or another cup of coffee, maybe a few more empty calories or some comforting sugar, and continually repeat this pattern until we take pills to fall asleep.

The mind has tricked us. We can't sleep, and the day repeats itself until it surrenders to exhaustion. The adrenal glands give up, the kidneys are now weakened, and the entire endocrine system is working overtime. Our immune systems work best when we are resting, but there's no rest with caffeine and sugar, so we never feel well, and always seem to have an allergy symptom, a cold, or aches and pains we can't get rid of. Our heart muscle is strained from the acid and the extra work, and our thyroids are overtaxed having to balance a metabolism that is stressed. Our backs ache more because we never really leave the day behind, and our feet hurt because we know, somewhere deep in our souls, that we're not on the right path. But, we take more pills, some that make us drowsy, others that warn us not to operate machinery or drive, and then order a pizza, an ice cream cone, or a loaded cheeseburger because, after all, we have to eat.

Finding the right food isn't that difficult. We are eighty percent water, so our food intake should be eighty percent alkaline. The twenty percent acid will be taken care of by the water we drink. The trick is to not play the supermarket game with coupons, specials, and discounts. Go directly to the produce aisles and stay away from all the others, except the grains and oils. Fruits and vegetables are abundant and meant to be the main course. Raw is best, steamed is okay, overcooked is a waste of time and money. Eat from the garden as you were meant to do. Remember that the heart chakra color is green so you want your food to harmonize. Broccoli, cucumber, kale, lettuce, parsley, green peas, green beans, zucchini, green apples, avocados, green onions, spinach, even dandelions and burdocks are the vegetables of choice. The green vegetables contain a balance of the nutrients our cells and tissues need to survive, one of the most important being vitamin A. This vitamin is an important antioxidant that enhances immunity, protects against pollution and cancer formation, and may also slow the aging process. We can't utilize protein without Vitamin A.

Green vegetables also contain many of the B complex vitamins, which should be taken together because they work as a team. When the entire team is utilized, we can add specific B's for various conditions. They are water soluble, which means they are excreted within four hours.

B1 is for the circulatory system and helps carbohydrate metabolism. It aids in muscle tone of the intestines and stomach. If you are taking contraceptives or sulfur drugs, or eat a high carbohydrate diet, you are probably lacking B1.

B2 is necessary for red blood cell formation and aids in the metabolism of carbohydrates, fats and proteins. It also helps tissues to use oxygen, so may help to improve your hair, skin and nails. Find it in asparagus, brussel sprouts, spinach, and broccoli.

B3 is for circulation and healthy skin. It lowers cholesterol and aids in the functioning of the nervous system. You'll find it in broccoli, but you'll have to add carrots, potatoes and tomatoes for this one.

B5 is the "antistress" vitamin and aids in the utilization of other vitamins. It helps the adrenal glands and aids in converting fats, carbohydrates and protein into energy. Without it, our adrenal glands become exhausted and we are constantly tired, nervous and depressed.

B6 is involved in more bodily functions than any other single nutrient. It is necessary in the production of hydrochloric acid for digestion and maintains the sodium and potassium balance needed by every cell. It is required by the nervous system and for the synthesis of RNA and DNA. These are the genetic instructions, much like computer programs, needed for the reproduction of all cells and for normal cellular growth. It inhibits the toxic chemical, homocysteine, which is an enemy of the heart muscle. It helps in treating asthma, arthritis and allergies. Find it in almost any food, but mostly in peas, spinach, carrots, avocado, beans, and cabbage.

B12 prevents anemia and nerve damage. It is required for proper digestion and fat metabolism. This is the one B vitamin not found in vegetables, so God did not intend us to be vegetarians. Cheese, eggs and seafood are the best sources of B12.

Biotin is a B vitamin, but you won't find many people lacking this nutrient as it is produced in the intestines from food. It aids in cell growth and in the utilization of the other B vitamins.

Choline is needed for nerve transmission, gallbladder and liver function, and aids in hormone production. Without this vitamin, brain and memory functions are impaired. You'll find this in egg yolks and whole grain cereals.

Folic acid is needed for energy production and red blood cell formation, but most importantly, helps regulate fetal development of nerve cells, vital for normal growth and development. Vegetables, bran, lentils, salmon, tuna and whole grains are the best sources.

Inositol is vital for hair growth and helps remove fats from the liver. Drinking coffee or caffeinated beverages will cause a shortage of this nutrient that is also found in vegetables, fruits, and whole grains.

Vitamin C is probably the best known and most talked about vitamin. What hasn't been talked about as much is the fact that Vitamin C needs Vitamin E to be most effective. Both are antioxidants, but they perform different functions. Vitamin E scavenges for dangerous oxygen radicals, and Vitamin C breaks them down. Most Vitamin C intake is lost in the urine and the body cannot manufacture this vitamin. We find it in vegetables, berries and citrus fruits. Aspirin, alcohol, smoking, antidepressants, and steroids reduce vitamin C levels in the body.

Vitamin D is the sun vitamin, and actually is not fully activated by food or supplements. It is vital for calcium and phosphorus absorption and necessary for normal growth and development of bones and teeth, especially in children. In fact, this vitamin supplement should not be taken without calcium. It's the sun vitamin, yet our schools have virtually eliminated the recess periods that allow children to play in the sun. Our fear of cancer keeps us from being in the sun, and we cover ourselves with lotions to protect us from its ultraviolet rays. Liver and gallbladder disorders interfere with its absorption, as do steroids and antacids. Fish oils, liver, salmon, tuna, alfalfa, and egg yolks contain some vitamin D. Osteoporosis is a common ailment, and people who have liver or kidney imbalances will not be able to absorb this important vitamin.

Vitamin E helps prevent cardiovascular disease and is a powerful antioxidant. It prevents cell damage and the formation of free radicals. It needs zinc to maintain proper levels in the blood, but should not be taken with iron. Dark, green, leafy vegetables and cold pressed vegetable oils are a vital source.

Vitamin K is needed for clotting, as God thought of everything when He created us, and is found in alfalfa, broccoli, cauliflower, cabbage, egg yolks, liver, oats and soybeans.

Vitamin P, or bioflavinoids, enhance Vitamin C absorption and should be taken together. The white material just beneath the peel in citrus fruits contains bioflavinoids, so we need to eat this part when we peel grapefruit, oranges, lemons and apricots. Bioflavinoids work synergistically with Vitamin C to protect the capillaries, the small blood vessels, and have an antibacterial effect. They promote circulation, stimulate bile production, lower cholesterol levels, and may prevent cataracts.

Minerals are also found in food and are naturally occurring in the Earth. The body stores minerals primarily in bone and muscle tissue, and they are competitive with each other and should be taken in balanced amounts. Zinc, for instance, can deplete copper if we take too much of it, and excessive calcium can deplete magnesium.

Calcium is not only important in the formation of strong bones and teeth, but also helps to maintain a regular heartbeat. It also protects the bones and teeth from lead, a toxic metal found in paints and the pipes of older homes. Boron is necessary for calcium absorption, and too much calcium can interfere with zinc absorption. Insufficient Vitamin D will inhibit calcium absorption as will excess phosphorus. Phosphorus is in soft drinks. Green, leafy, vegetables, kelp, sesame seeds, yogurt and cheese are good sources.

Copper aids in the formation of bone and red blood cells, and works in balance with zinc and calcium to form elastin. It's needed for a healthy nervous system, but its levels are reduced if we take too much zinc or vitamin C. The same is true in the reverse. If we absorb too much copper, our vitamin C and zinc levels will be reduced. Salt-water purifiers will often leech copper from house plumbing and may contribute to lower Vitamin C and zinc levels. Iodine, found in iodized salt, is important in trace amounts. It helps to metabolize fat, and is important for a healthy thyroid gland. Breast cancer has also been linked to a deficiency in iodine. We get copper from almonds, avocados, beans, garlic, oranges, and green, leafy vegetables.

Iron's primary function is the production of hemoglobin

and the oxygenation of red blood cells. Vitamin C increases absorption of iron, but we also must have sufficient hydrochloric acid in the stomach. Brittle nails, hair loss, fatigue and anemia all come from a deficiency in this mineral.

Magnesium assists in calcium and potassium absorption and is vital for nerve and muscle impulses. It helps prevent depression, heart disease and high blood pressure. We find this in dairy products, apples, bananas, green, leafy vegetables, whole grains, and seafood. Fluoride, found in most toothpaste and alcohol, and excessive amounts of zinc, deplete magnesium.

Manganese is essential, not only for those deficient in iron, but also for the utilization of B1 and Vitamin E. It's used for fat metabolism, healthy nerves, and a strong immune system. Avocados, nuts, seeds, and whole grains are the primary source.

Phosphorus is needed for bones and teeth, the heart muscle, and kidney function, and must be in balance with calcium and magnesium. Soda, or pop, depending on your area of the country, contains high amounts of phosphorus, which interferes with calcium absorption. Drink a dozen sodas and you'll be nervous, irritable, suffer bone loss, and not be able to sleep. Feed sodas to your children and increase the possibility of lead toxicity, nervousness, cavities, and eczema.

The heart and the nervous system need potassium. It also works with sodium to regulate the body's water balance. Diuretics, stress, and laxatives cause a potassium imbalance. Avocados, brown rice, bananas, raisins, potatoes and wheat bran are good sources.

Selenium, especially when combined with vitamin E, is a powerful antioxidant and helps to maintain a healthy heart. It is also vital to pancreatic function and tissue elasticity. Green, leafy vegetables, garlic, onions, salmon, tuna and whole grains are the best sources.

Silicon holds us together and is necessary for healthy

hair, skin, nails and arteries. It counteracts the effects of aluminum, of which fluoride is a by-product, and may prevent Alzheimer's and osteoporosis. Green, leafy vegetables, brown rice, peppers, and beets contain silicon. Sulfur is an acid-forming mineral that disinfects the blood and slows down the aging process. It helps to balance the Ph and protects us from pollution. Eggs, garlic, fish, onions, and cabbage are excellent sources.

Finally, zinc, found in fish, poultry, whole grains, liver, pecans, mushrooms and sunflower seeds, is vital in protecting the liver from chemical damage and promoting a healthy immune system; however, dosages of more than 100 milligrams can depress the immune system, and hard water consumption can disrupt the balance.

All of these need to work together as a team. Too often, we see the "miracle" vitamin or mineral being advertised or touted as the "one" you need. Though symptoms occur from depletion or excessive amounts, as we've illustrated, no one vitamin or mineral should be used or abused to "cure" a problem or condition. We need vitamin/mineral supplements because of air, water, and soil pollution, but these supplements need to be balanced, without the addition of herbs, sweeteners, or synthetic preservatives.

We don't need "junk" food, or fast food, or microwaved, or synthetic, or processed food. We need to rekindle our relationship to the Earth and its bounty. The Earth will provide, and if we follow the simple rule of eating only the amount we need, and stick to the natural abundance provided for us, we will reduce, possibly eliminate, a host of diseases and symptoms, and live a longer, happier, life.

Good food and healthy water, in balance. The first two keys to health.

CHAPTER VIII

The third vital key to staying in balance is breathing. This may sound too rudimentary to some, since we breathe every day, or so we think. The truth is, most Americans don't breathe at all. Check your breathing right now. Are you holding your breath? When you believe you are breathing, can you feel your breath all the way into your abdomen? Are you breathing through your nose or your mouth? Can you feel your diaphragm "massaging" your organs as you inhale and exhale?

When you truly breathe, you inhale life, and life is God. Polluted, toxic air obviously doesn't come from the Creator, and because we constantly exchange air with each other, with plants and animals, and within our organs and internal systems, we should be aware of what's in that air, and how to get the best air we can. God meant the air to be cleansed by the recycling of clean water, rejuvenated by photosynthesis, and inhaled deeply to oxygenate and fortify our bodies.

Nitrogen makes up 78% of the earth's atmosphere and is normally colorless, odorless, non-metal gas. It is a part of all living tissue. Nitric oxide, the compound of nitrogen and oxygen, maintains our cardiovascular, immune and central nervous systems. In fact, the enzyme that produces nitric oxide is abundant in the brain.

Nitrates and nitrites, normally naturally occurring parts of the nitrogen cycle, have been radically altered by the use of fertilizers, herbicides, and chemical production. Our soil and water tables are permeated with these compounds, which have a dangerous and adverse effect on the thyroid. They also cause a shortage of Vitamin A and are known carcinogens.

We don't readily use the nitrogen we breathe, as it is converted from the atmosphere and used by plants, which we then ingest. 20% of our atmosphere is oxygen, and this becomes our vital breathing link. The problem is, industrial air pollution, diesel fuels, and recycled polluted water and soil pollutants, have reduced the percentage of readily available oxygen. Our bodies will attempt to filter the air, through hair follicles, mucus membranes and water dilution, which is similar to the earth's defenses. Our natural defense on a physical, and perhaps, spiritual level, is to not breathe. This robs the body of the increasingly small amounts of oxygen it needs to maintain life. We are already losing the valuable properties of oxygen in our food and water.

The sensible thing to do is to give our bodies a fighting chance. By breathing deeply, we increase the percentage of available oxygen and increase our chances of utilizing oxygen in the formation of nitrous oxide. The physical process of breathing also is helpful to the body's balance. By fully expanding the chest and stretching the diaphragm, we are, in essence, "massaging" the vital organs that reside above and below this muscle. This increases circulation to these organs, while also delivering oxygen.

Hyperventilation is another problem and is caused by breathing too quickly. Again, we don't inhale enough oxygen, nor do we expel carbon dioxide and other toxic gases, which robs our tissues and cells of oxygen, causes dizziness and memory loss, and eventually destroys cellular walls.

Ionic air cleaners can help rid home and internal car environments of pollutants and maybe give us a better fighting chance to breathe, but the most important approach is to begin learning how to breathe in the life you've been given, with the faith that your body will either handle the pollutants because you have the nutrients and healthy water you need, or alert you so you can make changes.

These first three keys may seem too simplified or elementary to many people. Water, food, and air are not "miracle" cures, but are miracles themselves. We take them for granted and abuse them. We rely on synthetic material to nourish a body created with meticulous love and care, and complain about the cost of health care and pharmaceuticals. Except for the shelter we believe we need, these three keys are essentially free.

If you believe you can't afford healthy water, skip two meals or a golf outing and at least purchase filters for your drinking water and shower. Be scrupulous when deciding on which purification company provides what is necessary to properly filter water, and then do the work necessary to keep it running efficiently.

If you believe you can't find healthy food or don't have time to shop for it, just start at the fruit and vegetable aisle. Skip the meat, soda, beer, coffee and cigarettes, and you'll have more than enough for good salads, raw vegetable plates, stir-fries, and exotic rice dishes.

If you believe clean air is impossible, take some action to change it. Walk to work, or change jobs so you can. Force automakers to stop polluting your vital life force. Boycott industries that continue to ignore air regulations. Empower lawmakers to increase the standards of air quality. At the very least, provide yourself and your family with a reliable air cleaning system so you can breathe healthy air while you sleep. Again, skip a meal, a text message, or a new suit, and purchase an ionic air cleaner.

A passion for life is half the battle. Belief is the second half. These three keys are the outer circle of your earth walk.

CHAPTER IX

The fourth key you need to pick up and keep with you on your earth walk, is the walk itself. We are not furniture. We are living, vital miracles, meant to walk, run, climb, swim and play. As babies, we learn to crawl, and then beam with pride when our first steps are recognized. Barely confident in this new found pleasure, we see older children running, and we strive to catch up. It feels good. The more we run, jump, and play, the more we want to do it again.

In school, our physical education teachers were once our heroes. They could teach us to play all the games Mom, Dad, or the kids next door didn't know how to play. They taught us about the seemingly limitless powers our bodies have, and pushed us to physically find the spiritual warrior.

Our bicycles were our horses and we rode the wind. We climbed trees, swung on vines, skated, played baseball, basketball, and hide and seek. Not once did we use a mouse or a joystick to win or lose a game. Not once did we think of riding on a board, or motorizing our transportation. We walked. We ran. We moved our legs.

Summer time was playtime, and no mother in tune with the times allowed her children to stay inside. They knew we needed fresh air and sunshine. They knew we needed to stretch and exercise, and that we would enjoy doing it. Summer camp was something many children looked forward to and actually enjoyed. To many, it was the best time of their lives. They were one with nature and in tune with themselves, and they counted the last days of spring and of school in expectation of playing and being at camp.

What happened? How did we become car drivers with tired passengers? Why do we view sports as spectator gatherings and junk food galas? When did we decide air conditioned rooms were better than sweating in the fresh air? How did imagination become role-playing in a video game, rather than the joyful fantasizing of being a hero or just cloud walking to enjoy the day?

Every living thing on Earth stretches and moves, from snakes and toads, to trees, flowers and ants. Every creature and plant unspoiled by human attitude, knows it needs to move to continue living.

Trees have roots that reach into the pulse of the earth, but their branches call to the wind and they sway in its rhythm. Flowers open and close, dogs stretch and wag, birds spread their wings and sing. Humans grumble and stumble to the bathroom and coffee pot, read emails to catch up on the news, watch soap operas or reality shows to stimulate their brains, and do most of this while sitting in a car, on a train, or crooked on a couch.

Stretching hurts. Legs get cramps and backs spasm. Joints crack from too much carbon dioxide, and fallen arches from standing on concrete or wearing unsupportive shoes make our feet swell and hurt. Shoulders are constantly aching, and it hurts too much to stretch our arms over our heads. We can't touch our toes because our bellies are in the way, or our hamstrings are too tight, or our backs have too many fusions. We can't open like a flower, or reach high to sway in the wind, or even spread our wings to fly.

Ligaments and joints need fluid, oxygen, enzymes and nutrients. The circulatory system needs water, oxygen and movement to keep it strong and flexible. The lymphatic system, our immune system, needs muscle contraction to move metabolic waste out of our bodies. Muscles need nutrients, water and movement to stay supple and strong. Spines need water, nutrients and alignment to provide structure and nerve impulses for movement. Bones need oxygen, water, and minerals to help the muscles to move. The digestive system needs to be stretched and strengthened to allow for nutrient absorption and waste product disposal. Lungs need expansion and contraction to exchange bad air for good, and the heart needs healthy blood, water and minerals to maintain its beat, its connection to earth and God.

Yoga, tai chi, and Qi gong, are popular stretching and meditative exercises. Aerobics increase oxygen uptake and strengthen the heart, but too many of these programs fail to incorporate stretching before and after.

None of these exercises will be beneficial to the body, of course, unless there is proper nutrition and water consumption.

One of the most vital areas of our bodies that needs daily stretching is the back. The spine and its connection to the brain control every organ and system. It is dependant on water, as the intervetebral discs provide cushioning for our upright frames. The spine is an "S" curve, which keeps us upright and moves in unison with every twist and turn. When we turn our heads to the right or to the left, our lower back, the lumbar and sacral area, holds steadfast so we don't spin with the movement. When we take a forward step, the spine maintains an opposing force so we don't fall forward.

The back, leg, and neck muscles attach to our hips and shoulders, and to the spine, so they can coordinate our movements. Our nervous system is dependant on the alignment of the vertebrae in the spine, and thus the balance of energy within our bodies.

Chiropractors are trained to manipulate the vertebrae, sometimes too forcefully, but more often through soft tissue pressure. The art and science of this manipulation has been in existence for thousands of years. Chinese records from 2700 B.C. show some of the earliest manipulations, and the Greeks recorded leg manipulations to relieve lower back pain. In 1895, in the United States, Daniel Palmer first performed chiropractic manipulations on a patient who had been deaf for seventeen years after he felt something change in his back. After manipulating the spine in the upper back, the patient reported that his hearing improved.

What we don't realize or seem to remember, is that we can do many of the same manipulations performed by chiropractors through stretching. We did it as children. We rolled on the floor, brought our knees to our chests, curled into the fetal position, hung upside down from monkey bars, touched our toes without bending our knees, and did push-ups without raising our bellies from the floor. All of these movements have been copied by ancient practices, such as yoga, and helped our backs to remain aligned, strong, and supple.

Of course, as children, we also slept on smaller pillows, exercised more, drank more fluids, and ran on the earth, rather than on concrete. Children today are visiting the chiropractor more often, or worse, having back pain and back surgery because of sublaxations and misalignment. Poor nutrition, soda instead of water, lack of physical exercise, and poor posture are all contributing to the imbalances in our children. Since the spinal nerves connect to all other systems, children's diseases, physical and mental, are on the increase and the drug industry is flourishing.

More than seventeen million Americans suffer from asthma, approximately 5 million of them being children. The prevalence of asthma in children has increased more than sixty percent since 1982. We blame this on second hand cigarette smoke or increased urban populations. This is partially correct. Children can't breathe because their diaphragms don't expand

and their spines are misaligned. The misalignment interferes
with the impulses to the lungs, the liver, the intestines, and the
endocrine system. Everything in the air becomes an allergen
and triggers an asthma attack. They can't breathe because of
psychological or spiritual triggers, sending them into panic
attacks that the body is no longer able to cope with. Inhalers
filled with steroids and bronchial dilators are carried to school
with peanut butter sandwiches, candy and soda. Recess is a
hand-held video game and after-school activities are bus
riding, television, and computer chat rooms.

Adults can't breathe because our pillows and beds are too
soft, our diets are poor, our shoes (especially women's shoes),
don't support our spines, and we sit at desks or in car seats or
sideways on couches.

In the peripheral nervous system, which is made up of the
nerves that run from the brain and spinal cord, there are
chemical signals that pass between neurons and muscles or
glands. These transmitters either activate or inhibit cell
functions. ADHD, or attention deficit hyperactivity disorder,
is treated with drugs that alter the chemistry of these
transmitters, the belief being that the problem is in the brain
and that the electro-chemical processes need to be changed.
Nowhere in research studies is it suggested that spinal
alignment, along with proper nutrition, including healthy
water, could be the answer to the behaviors associated with
ADHD. In other words, children could be hyperactive, because
they are not active.

Animals, except those in unhealthy, domesticated
environments, don't have asthma or ADHD, although many
animals are now starting to suffer from environmental and
water pollution. Most animals have straighter spines that don't
need to support the weight as humans do, but they still stretch,
exercise, and try to drink clean water.

The spine, spinal nerves, and nerve processes don't need to
be fused or surgically altered. They need to be open to allow
the electrical impulses necessary for life.

Before you move from your bed in the morning, freeze in your waking position and check how you are lying on your pillow. Does it support your neck, or is your arm providing the support? Is your bed too soft or too hard so that your legs or back ache even before you put weight on them? Do you always sleep on one side of the bed, or roll to one side because of a partner? These things alter the alignment of your spine and need to be changed.

Before you get up, stretch. Lay flat and bend your knees. Cross one leg over the other so the heel is on the knee forming a triangle, and rock your leg. This helps to open the hip joint and break down calcium deposits formed from inactivity or inflammation. Straighten the leg and make wide circles in both directions to open the entire ball and socket joint that will be supporting you throughout the day.

Bend your leg and bring the knee to your chest using a towel or strap and pulling your foot toward you. If you use your hands, you are also using your back muscles and more than likely twisting your upper torso. Use a towel and pull your knee as close to your chest as you can. Hold it there for a moment and feel the stretch in your lower back and buttocks.

Now straighten that same leg again, locking the knee and pointing the toes toward the ceiling. Slide the towel behind your ankle and breathe in deeply. When you exhale, pull that leg over your head and hold it there. Your hamstrings will probably hurt, but not forever.

Do the same routine with the other leg and know that you are helping your lower back get ready for the day. When you are finished, slide the towel behind both ankles and pull both legs over your head. This helps the sacrum to readjust.

Sit up and place the towel behind your neck. Keep your back and shoulders straight and let your chin fall to you chest. After a moment, pull the towel a little and feel the stretch in the cervical vertebrae in your neck.

Now you're almost ready to stand up and allow your blood to flow. Have a glass of water first. Those little sponges called intervetebral discs have "dried" out a little during your sleep. Water them so they can cushion your stance and help you to stay aligned.

You've stretched many of the muscles that will keep you upright. Though not a complete stretching routine, it's a start. Many other muscles will be stretched on your earth walk.

You are "plugged in" and normal body processes are now freer to perform the functions they were intended to perform. Get up on your toes and stretch your arms high over your head. Sway in the wind or soar like a bird. Walk, and know that walking is a gift. Run, and feel the wind. This, too, is a gift. Do these things with your children and your friends and know that you are giving them the gift of alignment and movement, the freedom to be human, the power of the fourth key to balanced health.

CHAPTER X

W hat we take into our bodies must be processed, utilized, or eliminated. The healthy, though somewhat complicated, path of digestion and elimination is the fifth key to balanced health.

Our digestive systems are roughly thirty feet long and include the mouth, salivary glands, stomach, liver, gallbladder, pancreas and intestines. Picture a long, curved tube from your mouth to your anus. Because we can't utilize food in its dense form, the salivary glands in our mouth secrete digestive enzymes to begin to break down the food into carbohydrates, fats, and protein. Once we begin to swallow, the nervous system is triggered to continue the push down the esophagus to the stomach.

The stomach basically has three functions. The first is to store the food we eat because the digestive process is not instantaneous. The upper part of the stomach relaxes to allow for this storage. Digestive enzymes from the pancreas and hydrochloric acid are mixed with the food to continue breaking it down, which also allows the lower part of the stomach to empty the contents into the small intestines. The liver produces bile and stores it in the gallbladder until the brain triggers the gallbladder to release it into the bile ducts and then into the small intestine when we eat. These bile acids break down fats, which is why many people have trouble avoiding weight gain after gallbladder removal. The fats are then digested by pancreatic enzymes and the small intestine.

Glucose, a product of carbohydrate digestion, is carried through the bloodstream to the liver where it is stored or used for energy.

Proteins are large molecules that need pancreatic and stomach enzymes, along with enzymes from the small intestine, to convert them to amino acids. The amino acids are then absorbed through the intestinal walls into the bloodstream and transported to all parts of the body for cellular growth and repair.

Fats are a large source of energy and go through several stages of transformation before their storage or utilization in all parts of the body.

This process takes anywhere from three to six hours. Everything left over from this process, usually undigested food and watery juices, gets moved to the large intestine, which is the colon. Finally, the material consisting of undigested food, water, salts, bacteria and mucus are moved to the rectum and stored until we eliminate them.

How many meals do you eat a day and how large are they? How often do you eliminate the toxic materials from your body? How often do you stretch and massage your abdominal area? How much do you dilute the digestive enzymes necessary for this process by drinking fluids with food? The stomach lining is protected from the effects of hydrochloric acid, but not from other acids. Other organs utilize some acids, but are not protected from the effects of hydrochloric acid. How many times do you swallow antacids before or after a meal?

Your central nervous system provides triggers for the secretion of gastric juices. How do you sit when you eat? Is your spine and nervous system aligned and working correctly to aid you in your digestive process?

The liver absorbs alcohol and drugs, chemically treating them to rid the body of poisons. If you are on medications and drinking alcohol with your meal, how much are you taxing this vital organ?

With all of this in mind, we move to the colon. We consider this organ a "waste depository" and take it for granted. Colon cancer is one of the biggest killers, yet we ignore the colon until it's too late. The colon and the liver have an obvious relationship in digestion, with the liver acting as a protector and defender against toxic chemicals and waste. If the colon isn't healthy, the liver can't perform and the blood becomes toxic, which affects every organ.

The ascending, transverse and descending colon contain "maps" to every system and organ in the body. The brain is in constant communication with the colon, not only providing signals, but also receiving feedback on what is being left behind and eliminated. In simplest terms, the colon takes inventory and may tell the brain it didn't digest vitamin A or some of the fats or sugars necessary for survival. The brain then checks with other organs to see if they have received their vital nutrients. Each organ reports back, and if there is something lacking, the brain may trigger a craving or a thirst, telling us something is out of balance. The colon receives all of this information and compiles it. It sends nerve impulses back to each organ and verifies the information.

If we don't eliminate the toxins from the colon, the undigested food putrefies and begins to release gases. These gases ferment and become toxic to the mucosal walls, eventually seeping into the bloodstream, and always going through the liver.

The colon has registered which organs have received the nutrients it needs for growth and survival and maintains this record in its cell memory. All of the organs and systems, through the brain, register their strength or weakness in the iris of the eye. The central nervous system also compiles a list of organs that are not responding to stimuli and stores this list in the eyes and the memory of the colon. Western medicine may view this as unscientific because the body's miraculous complications make it too difficult to test and retest all theories under a microscope, but those who understand the energy of this system know the colon must be clean and cleansed of debris, bacteria and parasites for the body to be healthy

Picture A

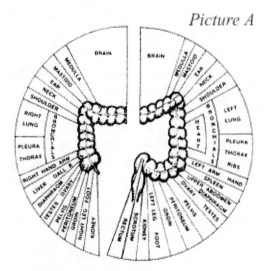

*Bowel chart indicating reflex reference
to the organs in the iris*
By Dr. Bernard Jensen, USA

    The colon's structure can be compared to a galvanized pipe, much like those used for decades in our sewer systems. Repeated sludge and slow movement blocks the pipe and less material is able to move through smoothly. Add dehydration or no water to the equation and we have a very backed up cess pool harboring dangerous bacteria and disease, no longer able to receive waste, respond to or interact with the small intestine or the brain.

Why can't we let go? We take in food and water, but we also take in energy. If someone says we're fat or ugly or dumb or too short, we have a hard time digesting it. If we fear rejection, or judge others, which is self-judgment reflected, we can't digest it. The liver tries to help, as one of its more than five hundred jobs is to hold anger and resentment and try to convert it. The energy is the same negative frequency of poisons, and the liver struggles. If we don't exercise and move, rejuvenate the lymphatic system, the fats stored in the lymph begin to clog and multiply, expanding with every meal and seeping into the circulatory system. The poor heart, just a beating muscle to scientists, takes on some of the burden of the fat and cholesterol as it weeps for us, and the colon screams with congestion. We don't let go. We hold onto our fears and in our attempt to control life or the lives of others, we end up controlling our bowels.

The toxins continue to build and to permeate every tissue and every cell. The vibrational energy emanating from us becomes negative, dark and dense. As each organ reports that it no longer is receiving the life-giving nutrition it needs, the section of the colon that contains that file begins to shut down. The colon itself is sick, and it transmits that illness to our entire being.

This is a prolapsed colon with indicators in the iris.

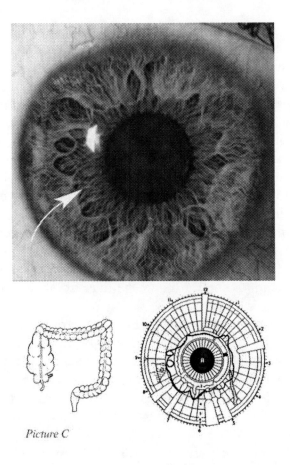

Picture C

Colon cancer, liver cancer and heart disease. The three biggest killers in the United States. Let go! Tell your ego to take a hike and stop trying to live everyone else's life but your own. You are not in charge. You have a duty to maintain your body as a harbor for your soul. That's your job. Your colon needs to know that the digestive system as a whole has received the needed nutrients, and that all systems are working. It needs to hear from every organ that all is well so the brain can trigger its release. It needs the vibrations of fruits, vegetables and water to remove the sludge and make it hum like a well-cared-for car.

Physically and physiologically, colon hydrotherapy can help. However, cleansing the colon will do nothing if you continue to feed it garbage, and garbage is emotional, mental, chemical, and electrical,

Fasting is a good place to start an overall cleansing program that will especially help the liver and colon. Fasting is not starvation. Pick two days when you can maybe be alone so you can "go within." Drink your morning water, do your stretches, play music that resonates with your soul, and walk your medicine wheel.

Three to four times the first day, drink water with fresh lemon added. This helps the liver to release more toxins and can aid in breaking down calcium deposits that can form stones. Always follow this with more water thirty minutes later to wash the acid from your teeth. The teeth, by the way, are a very important link to our systemic health. Cracks under crowns can allow bacteria into our circulatory system. Poor hygiene not only allows bacteria to accumulate between teeth, but also penetrates the mucus membranes in the mouth, and therefore becomes part of the food we're tying to digest. Dental amalgams, fillings, seep metals into our bodies through these same mucus membranes, and we should consider replacing them to cleanse these metals from our systems. We check the teeth on horses, brush our pet dog's teeth, and know that unsightly smiles are not something we want, but we forget about the health of our teeth and mouths, and how important this is in the overall scheme of balanced health.

At noon, drink a large glass of fresh vegetable juice. Before retiring, drink three to four ounces of Aloe Vera juice, preferably George's. The aloe soothes inflamed organs and tissues.

On the second day, follow the same routine, but at noon drink a large glass of fresh fruit juice, preferably apple juice as the pectin helps to remove heavy metals from the organs. Before retiring, drink a smaller glass of vegetable juice to replenish vitamins and minerals.

On the third day, you no longer have to fast, but you should add foods sensibly and in small quantities. Begin with water and the usual routine. Eat fruit such as an apple and some blueberries, and after thirty minutes, add a whole grain cereal. Get back on your liquid vitamins and minerals and add liquid acidophilus to replace the good intestinal flora that you may have eliminated. For lunch and dinner, have raw or lightly steamed vegetables alone or with brown rice.

Repeat this menu on the fourth day and you should be seeing consistent bowel movements and begin to feel a little lighter. The average amount of built up, stored fecal matter in humans is anywhere from fifteen to twenty-five pounds. You'll lose a little water weight, but your goal is to cleanse the colon of this rotten debris.

On the fifth day, have oatmeal or another grain cereal for breakfast, but try to avoid the processed, sugary stuff. Also, try to avoid milk as it increases mucus and slows the cleansing process. Apple juice on cereal actually tastes good, and again, the pectin helps eliminate metals. Eat some raw vegetables such as broccoli, carrots, cauliflower and celery for lunch, and for dinner some more steamed vegetables including yellow onions, and garlic over brown rice.

Five days to begin cleaning a lifetime of sludge shouldn't be too hard. If you feel hungry, know you are more likely thirsty and drink water. If you have trouble sleeping, have a cup of herb tea before bed. If you are still feeling constipated, increase your water intake and on the next day add more fiber. Though you're not rid of the intestinal parasites or Candida that has probably set up housekeeping in your digestive tract, you have a cleaner path to start dealing with those particular problems, and your liver and colon may be strong enough to handle whatever healing regimen you decide on.

Repeat the fast within four to six weeks, but this time on the third day add more grapefruit, and on the fourth and fifth days, add herbs that will go after parasites. We all have parasites of one kind or another, but when our digestive tracts are sluggish, or we have a build up of yeast, or our immune systems are depressed, opportunistic parasites and worms can make your entire body ill.

I first learned about colon health in 1976, at a retreat in upstate New York. A chiropractor who did high colonic therapy had a patient who experienced epileptic seizures. At the time, doctors wanted to medicate or operate, but the patient's father knew there were alternatives and supported his daughter's therapy. It took several weeks of colonics, diet changes, massage and psychological support, but the end result was nothing short of amazing. The colonic revealed dead and rotting worms that had been embedded in the walls of the ascending colon. That particular area of the colon sends electrical impulses to report on conditions in the brain and nervous system. When the worms were eliminated, the patient had a full recovery and came back twenty years later to testify on the benefits of colonic therapy. She never had another seizure.

We get intestinal parasites from meats, water, even animal kisses on the nose, and if our systems are acidic or otherwise conducive to harboring these invaders, they will set up shop, and they'll populate as many weakened areas as they can find. They travel in lymph fluids and in the blood, so can cause imbalance in any organ or tissue.

Parasites also thrive in yeast. We all have yeast, a living organism that normally lives in a benign state within our bodies. One species, Candida Albacans, can multiply and cause extreme conditions, especially when influenced by antibiotics and depressed immune systems. When left untreated, the yeast will spread through the bloodstream to other organs and act like a magnet for bacteria, fungus and mold. Difficult to get rid of, but not impossible. Its elimination is vital in colon and digestive health.

The important thing to remember is that your colon, gallbladder, liver, stomach and pancreas have to be clean and strong enough to go through a parasite or yeast cleanse, so take it one step at a time.

Another important thing to remember is the lesson of the clogged colon and/or parasite invasion. We have to be clear about our boundaries, both physically and emotionally. We allow parasites in the form of friends or community to sap our energy and destroy our balance. We allow learned judgment and fears to fill us with matter and organisms not reflective of or conducive to our growth as loving, human beings. Set your boundaries, with love and not fear. Form your circle and become the great mystery in the middle, the fire, the beginning of everything. Find your passion from the miracles around you. Find your truth and your faith. Faith, trust, an inner knowing that you're okay and you'll be okay will set you free. Then fill your heart and your body with all that is good and good for you. You'll be able to let go, and you'll hold the fifth key to health.

CHAPTER XI

Your mind is very powerful, and also very weak. Because we have such confusion about the mind, we are never sure if it is our minds that are speaking, our hearts, or just the idle words of others. We don't know if we think with our minds, and then translate our thoughts, or if our unconscious mind does the thinking, and then we distort the thought with our learned experience.

Trust comes from the mind, faith from the heart. We trust or distrust all that we know and all that we don't know. The conscious mind takes in the world and from whatever entry point, be it the eyes, the ears, the skin, or the memory, translates and discerns. Because we train the conscious mind, it too often does not check with the heart and the soul. Belief becomes a thought instead of a feeling, an argument instead of a given. What we believe, we will be, and it is because of this that we need to focus on the mind in all of its shapes and energies, to understand its connection to our bodies and our spirits. It is, after all, one significant part of the triangle, one third of the trinity.

The mind is also a triangle. The conscious, sub-conscious, and unconscious are each a powerful leg. We are most familiar with the conscious, as this is our reality, our present, or so we believe. We are conscious of our wants and desires, of our dislikes and likes, of our behavior, our needs, and our existence.

Yet our conscious minds deceive us. What we believe we want is not always what was intended. What we believe to be acceptable behavior is not always accepted by others. What we think we need, we don't. Even our existence comes into question when we don't know our path.

What others tell or show us, we often take into our subconscious, and from there the energy, the frequencies of experience and memory, distort the picture, the sound, the reality and the truth, tossing out random bits of information and influencing our conscious awareness.

We hear we are old, and therefore, unable to perform. Our subconscious mind translates the words from memory and experience, formats them into a belief, and sends the energy back to our conscious selves. Now we feel old. We "know" we can't perform. We trust that their observation of our present, conscious self, is truth. Our subconscious has reflected their judgment, their energy, and we have absorbed that energy into every cell, every organ, and every human part of us. The mind and the body have become a team, with the mind as the manager, and the body obeys.

Because we are human and give our conscious and sub-conscious minds such power, our spirit, the God within us, must also succumb. We are denied nothing. If we believe we are old, we will be, because we have a choice. Free will is the choice between good and evil, but what we choose to believe is what makes our human experience exactly that.

The God within us resides in our unconscious. Our deepest dream state, our attachment to the soul, our very spirit is within the unconscious. It has to be. Because we have free will, choice, and we are human, our spirit and soul must not be a part of our indecisions, judgments, and self-destruction. Because it is God, it can only be present where there is love, and the energy of unconditional intention.

Our conscious mind is one of opposites. Because we have choice, we must have answers. Yes or no, this way or that way, yin and yang. It also has three parts, three chambers. One chamber takes everything in, another expels unusable energy, and the third filters information from the subconscious.

Should we eat the ice cream, or not? Our subconscious remembers a time when ice cream made us feel better, made us feel loved. Our conscious mind knows that we decided yesterday to avoid ice cream so we can lose weight. Yes or no, no or yes? Our subconscious calls on spirit to help answer the question. "Are you coming from love or fear?" spirit asks. We love ice cream, but we're afraid that eating it will cause more weight gain. We love ice cream because we want and need to be loved, and eating ice cream reminds us of a time when someone did love us. They showed their love with an ice cream cone, and we believed we felt better.

"Then aren't you really coming from fear?" spirit asks.

Because we are afraid we're not loved, and we don't feel good about that, our conscious and unconscious mind is on its own. We now have a choice. We can choose to avoid the ice cream and stick to our conscious plan of trying to lose weight. Or we can choose to ignore the plan, and believe or trust that the ice cream will make us feel better. Spirit, our unconscious, is no longer involved, because we are still coming from fear.

If you choose the ice cream because you believe it will make you feel better, it will. For a while. But, you haven't faced the fear that began the desire for ice cream in the first place. You will still remember a time when someone loved you, and still feel the pain of not being loved as you believe, and another day will come when ice cream becomes a decision again.

Your body, in the meantime, has been passive in this decision. The choice that came from fear will eventually cause the body to react with the same negative energy. The fat from the ice cream won't be converted or processed, becoming more fat to be stored, and when you consciously realize you haven't lost weight, the question of whether you are loved will return.

It seems like a vicious cycle, but it doesn't have to be. The conscious mind can be retrained, and the sub-conscious can be reprogrammed, but you have to do the work.

The sixth key to balanced health is the retraining and reprogramming of these two areas of the mind, and one of the main ways of approaching this is with energy.

As we have said so often, we are energy. Everything we eat, drink, say, and think, is energy and has a frequency. Everything we take in, and everything we expel, is energy. We have negative and positive flow, and swirls of electromagnetic energy all around us. To change our minds, we have to change our energy. To change our energy, we need consistency, courage and a little bit of cosmic awareness.

Beyond the vibrational forces of the chakras, there exist layered, interactive waves of potential and actual energy. We are not just energy, but we emanate, reflect, and reciprocate energy. We are rainbows, but we are able to see rainbows only because their vibrations are dense enough for the human eye. The rainbows are everywhere and always around us, but their ethereal qualities and frequencies are not detected by the average human.

Our energy fields are multi-faceted and multi-dimensional. Our physical body is the densest energy we perceive, and has the lower vibrational frequencies.

Our etheric energy is the emanation that surrounds the physical body and holds the blueprint or master plan for every organ and cell. This energy is not a result of our physical selves, but rather the "parent." It is God's energy through thought manifested in the streaming, wavy pool of creation. Each thought is unique, each multiple set of vibrations different from any other. It is through this ethereal layer that we experience physical touch, hear words, see objects, smell odors, and react.

Our emotional energy is our personality, our outward eminence. E- motion, or energy in motion. It is the center of give and take, action and reaction.

Our mental energy is tri-fold, and is in constant interaction with our emotional, ethereal, physical energy closest to our body, and with our spiritual energy emanating the furthest from the physical and at the higher or highest frequencies. Of course, beyond this, there is Divine energy, which is the Creator or God, and we are human because we react to that energy. Seven energies coming from one, and one creating seven.

Because we have been trained to perceive our world three dimensionally and linearly, our energy is focused on the lower vibration of the physical. Those in some healing professions have been able to retrain themselves to experience the ethereal energy on some levels and will often refer to themselves as "energy healers." They practice Reiki, Quantum touch, touch for health, and other energy modalities. Because ethereal energy is the template for the physical, manipulating or massaging this energy can bring it into harmony, thus affecting the balance of the related organ or system within the body.

Because emotional energy directly affects the ethereal layer, we cannot have true healing without also dealing with the emotion behind the imbalance. We love ice cream because we reacted to someone loving us through the giving of ice cream. Because we are human and thrive on love, indeed, can't exist without it, our emotions recognize this as positive energy. Our ethereal body feels the emotional energy, but also "knows," because it harbors the master plan, that the ice cream can be negative to the physical, not because ice cream is "bad" for us, but because we are reacting to ice cream in a negatively emotional way.

Each energy field affects all of the others, and all of them affect each one. Again, this may sound complicated because we don't think beyond our human dimensions. To most of us, everything is linear. Time is on a line with a beginning and an end, electrons travel in perfect circles around a steadfast atom, our bodies have a top, bottom, front and back, and energy is somewhere inside of us.

To change our health, we have to change our energy, and to change our energy, we have to change our minds. Thoughts create, as proven by our existence. Thoughts create words, and spoken words also create.

God said, "Let there be light."

Emotions are either positive or negative; therefore come either from fear or from love. As simple as it may sound, we need to think love. Not the verb or act of love, but the noun, the being of love. We need to think, and therefore believe, that we love ourselves. That means we have adoration for what God has created, passion for the path of that creation, which is life. Every moment, awake or asleep, we need to think and manifest love. This is not yet spirit energy, but mental. If you are thinking at this moment that what was just said is silly, too simple, not real, impossible, ridiculous, and ludicrous or nonsense, then stop reading. Examine why your emotional energy caused your mental energy to come to these conclusions.

Loving ourselves is the hardest human undertaking. It means releasing and letting go of all things negative, and realizing that all those things come from fear. You are a victim, because Mom died when you were a baby, Dad tried to molest you, your brother beat you up, your boss fired you. You weren't tall enough, smart enough, fast enough, pretty enough. You didn't have money, or good clothes, or an education. You made wrong choices, but someone else made you choose. The all-inclusive "they" caused everything bad to happen to you. Because you maintain the victim's energy, you can't move forward. You're afraid of being a victim again. You're afraid making changes will cause more things to happen, and that you'll be the cause. How can you love yourself when you're sure no one else does? How can you forgive all the hurt, all the injustice, all the anger, when you can't forgive yourself?

Recognize that the initial fear, the most powerful fear to overcome, is the fear of change. Change is a word and a constant. If we fear change, we waste healing and loving energy on something that always is. The trick is to change for the better, and to have the courage to make changes. It isn't difficult. We all want to be better. We all, at one time or another, strive for perfection. Our souls give us direction. Our minds are our nemesis.

Begin each day with gratitude for the life you have, no matter how hard you believe it has been or it is. Stop being a victim of your life and choices. Begin each day loving, truly loving, the person in the mirror. Look at her or him as a parent looks at a child, with total, unconditional love.

As parents, we know our children will break the rules. We know they may try to lie, will think about stealing, will do things for attention, but we love them anyway. We don't condone such behavior. We, instead, guide them to change the way they look at things, the way they react to circumstances, and help them to discover new attitudes, insight and discernment.

Your inner child needs the same kind of parent, one that stops you from making the world a negative place and helps you find the good in everything around you.

My back was broken in an automobile accident. My first reaction was anger because the driver who caused the accident was inebriated. My anger turned to hatred and then to a willingness to do harm. All of these emotional reactions happened in an instant. Then I took back my energy, my power. Though the other driver was impaired and shouldn't have been driving, it was my energy that put me in her path. I had decided to take a different route home because I was tired and bored with my routine. My subconscious remembered many times in the past when I felt alone, used, over tired and sad because I had to work and always had to drive the same way home. My emotions were exacerbated by the memory of home being empty, and the fear that I would always be alone, always have to work, always have to drive the same way, be on the same path. I took a right turn instead of a left and put myself in the path of someone whose energy was also on a collision course. The negative vibration of my anger ballooned into the perceived emotion of hatred, and then to the potential of violence. I was afraid my back injury would keep me from working and afraid that not working would cause financial problems and other hardships in the future. All of this energy churned around me just before, during, and just after the accident.

The good in all of this? I volunteered with organizations that work to stop drunk driving. I learned more about back injuries and the healing alternatives to surgery. I also found a new way home from work. I learned about my temper, its origins, and learned how to change my reactions. I learned more about judgment. The drunk driver had just learned of her son's death, and though she never drank before, had a drink before going to identify the body. She was impaired, and crossed the line, but she had her own energy to learn from. I initially judged her as being irresponsible, negligent and "no good," when it was my judgment that was truly irresponsible. My fear and the energy that surrounded it had obscured my compassion, and my past, unrecognized, negative emotions, had made me fearful of the future.

All energy affects all energy, within us, around us, from us and to us.

Make a list of everything good about you, everything you love about you. Write it down, and then speak it. Make another list of everything you love about your parents, your kids, your spouse or partner. Write it, and then speak it, first to yourself, later to each of them. Make another list of everything you love about life and living. Write it, and then speak it. Say all of these things every day. Add to it as your thoughts create more good. Every time a negative thought tries to enter your mind, erase it and replace it.

The beginning of changing your energy so you can heal is changing the way you love yourself. With time, work, and patience, the conscious and sub-conscious mind will begin to believe you and the vibrational energy of love will increase and transform your emotional energy. As you continue, these energies will also affect the etheric energy, harmonizing and attuning the blueprint, the master plan. Our bodies strive for balance, for harmony, for healthy well-being. The etheric self longs for the frequency of unconditional, self-love. The physical body reacts to the symphony, absorbing the higher vibration, and in concert with nutrition, water, air, and movement, begins to heal itself. You have the sixth key

CHAPTER XII

"The first peace, which is the most important, is that which comes within the souls of people when they realize their relationship, their oneness with the universe and all its powers, and when they realize that at the center of the universe dwells the Great Spirit, and that this center is really everywhere, it is within each of us."

Black Elk, Native American

The spirit connection to our health is and is not a separate reality, a separate energy. It is the top of the pyramid, the energy with the highest potential. There is nothing that is not spirit, but when we speak of spirit and the mind-body connection, we have to first see the difference between the human spirit and that spirit which is considered divine.

All living things are endowed with spirit. They were created by God, or the Great Creator, and were created with intention. The immortal, non-physical essence of humans, apart from their intelligence or mind, is the human soul. We were spoken and breathed into being, and then connected to mind and body.

A bird has a spirit and a soul, though the brain or mind of a bird has less potential or capability than that of a human. The Earth is a living entity filled with animal, nature and human spirit, but also without a mind that must choose between perceived good and evil. Our spirit keeps us connected to God, while our mind is the separation.

In many religions, the separation from God is given a name and/or an identity. Christians believe in Satan, a devil, non-Godly being who dwells in Hell, an underworld hole where sinners are never forgiven. Eastern religions speak of a dark, fiery place where evildoers wait for judgment, much like a prison before a trial. In traditional native America, there is no Hell. We are, instead, one with the universe and with God, and know that God to be unconditional love. That love is a profound energy without boundaries or constraints, without judgment or punishment. We are beings and allowed to be. We are children, creations of a higher spirit, a greater creator, and strive to resonate with that vibration. It is within that energy that we begin to define the human soul.

I have been hit by lightning three times, survived earthquakes, blizzards and hurricanes. The power of the earth coupled with the moon and the stars is awesome and miraculous. I have cut the umbilical cord to unleash the wonder of new life, and held the hands of the dying while their spirits drifted away. I have ridden the waves of powerful oceans, cupped birds in my hand, assisted in the birth of kittens and puppies, and nursed a horse back to health. Thunder still drums visions into my heart, and rain on a Sunday morning in summer still rocks me into fetal position. Every day is a breath of life, every night a gentle kiss to sleep. Stars remind me of friends and family, and ducks flying South stir the wind under my own wings. I cry at sentimental commercials, laugh with my inner child, talk to trees and ants and rainbows as if they were long lost lovers, and marvel at mockingbirds singing the dew off the grass in the morning. My spirit is always with me. My human spirit. That amazing source of energy that surrounds my memory, my senses and my body.

Within that energy is a tiny part of God, filled with love, good intention, and childlike wonder. If God was the ocean and we dipped a thimble to fill it to the brim, we would have all the same ingredients, the same power and love, but in a much smaller amount. The essence in that thimble is your soul, the thimble itself your presence on Earth. Your human spirit is all that pours from the thimble while you're here on your earth walk. Your divinity is your eternal connection to that ocean.

We have within us and around us the power to re-create our lives, our health, and our intentions. We were whispered into existence with divine love, and every parent knows that once that whisper breathes and opens its eyes, we truly know what love is, and that love is unconditional. What mother would tempt her child with perils and misfortunes, and then send her into fire forever when she failed? What father would ask the impossible of his son, and then punish him for eternity when he didn't succeed? Love cannot create hell or damnation, but those who have proclaimed themselves the keeper of our spirits strive to convince us otherwise. Religion is not necessarily spirituality, but rather institutionalized codes, morals, tenets and practices. Organized religion has many forms and denominations, some of them exclusive of the existence of a God or a higher deity, but all based on an element of faith in some higher form of energy. The codes and ethics of organized religion more often than not use fear to convey their messages, and to ensure obedience from their congregations. The fear of going to a hellish place if one does not adhere to the specific codes of a church, or the belief that women have no divine presence in the universe, are examples of fear-driven religion useful only to those who seek power over the masses.

You are the keeper of your soul, and it is your relationship with your creator and the world He created for you that is your life. No fear can exist in that love, as no fear should exist in any relationship gifted with devotion.

When we feel that relationship, and know in our hearts that we have that love, our spirit is strong and our bodies always ready to be lifted in that energy. Healing and the ability to heal are inherent in our relationship to spirit. Our body's purpose is to harbor the soul while it dances through the maze of its mission. Everything we see, touch, hear, smell and remember has spirit, but once our soul is surrounded by our human selves, our minds forget and cause us to believe that we are no longer of God, with God, a part of God. We spend our embodied lives searching for that connection in churches, synagogues, religious texts and rituals. The truth is the connection was never lost. God, spirit, has always been and will always be with us. That's why we have sunsets and moonrises, stars that twinkle and wink, and clouds that play hide and seek with the light. It's always there, but you have to be open enough, brave enough, loving enough to see it and to know it. That "knowing" is a part of your healing, a necessary energy for your balanced health. Stop believing in someone else's miracle vitamin or cure. Stop listening to infomercials and drug commercials that lure you into more imbalance, more illness. If you listen with your mind, you will be deceived. Listen instead with your heart, your intuition, your soul. Feel your connection to the earth, but more importantly, your connection to your creator. When you know something is wrong with your ear or your knee or your teeth, ask. Ask through that wonderful spirit within you. Ask your spirit-self to help you find the answer. If you've done the work, the answer will come, because the question is the answer. Because spirit is within you, you already know. But you have to believe you deserve to be well. You have to believe you are strong enough, wise enough, divine enough to heal yourself. And you are.

The medical establishment has been trained to do the best they can, but only with each other's conclusions. Many of them do care, and they do want you to get well, but their resources are tied to pharmaceutical and insurance companies, and their licenses are constantly threatened with litigation. Their education, until recently, has been rigidly tied to archaic practices and a belief system that only they know the answer to your body's condition, and therefore, the future of your soul. A doctor who has studied the results of tests endorsed by insurance companies and validated by the research of their colleagues, is only as good as the one who invented the test. You, on the other hand, have lived your entire life within the context of your present problem. You have all the research within reach, and the only colleague you need is within you.

Of course, we need physicians in emergencies and for surgeries caused by neglect and self-abuse. The first doctors were surgeons, and that remains their specialty. Your specialty is self. No one knows your history, your habits, your "keys" as you do. No one can experience your pain, your symptoms, the same way you do. Your etheric energy contains the master program, and your spirit knows the code.

Your spirit, your soul, is the seventh key. It is your belief system, the system that rules all others. If you believe you have cancer, or that eating spaghetti will cause you to contract cancer, or that cancer will kill you, that belief will become a reality. Spirit, God, will not deny you. Because you are human, you have free will and choice.

"Ask, and it shall be given you; seek, and you shall find; knock and it shall be opened unto you. For every one that asketh, receiveth; and he that seeketh, findeth; and to him that knocketh it shall be opened. [Matthew 7:7-8]."

How do you ask? How do you connect with God? Over two billion people believe we need to go to a building, kneel, obey the priest's words and tell ourselves we are sinners. Another 180 million people believe in the synagogue as the place of refuge and redemption. Still more believe in mosques and a reward in heaven for doing the deeds of leaders. We are the direct connection between heaven and earth. We are the conduits of light and energy. We are the heartbeat of God. No building or code of conduct or textbook or moral reference manual will bring you closer to God. Indeed, these things more often than not will move people to judgment, anger, hatred and violence because they are not truly based in love, but stagnated

FORGET THE CURES FIND THE CAUSE

in fear. We were given rules of life, very basic rules, translated and re-interpreted, but still the rules from our parent. They are simple, and even children recognize them as being easy to follow. When we follow the basic rules, our spirits are free, and God is no longer an energy to be feared, but a divinity to be loved without question.

My little girl was four or five when we heard a radio newscast about a flogging that was to occur because some teenage boys damaged automobiles in another country. They were wrong, but the flogging was based on the belief that harsh punishment was just, whether the teenagers died or not. When I turned off the newscast, the little soul sitting next to me said, "Gee, I'm glad we have rules." When I asked her what she meant by that, she said, "Well, we have seven or ten rules. That's all. And if we follow the rules, we're free to do everything else."

The simplicity and truth in her words was God-like, and I was reminded to come to God as a child, and to be God-like in my parenting of my own child. That little girl has grown into a woman who has never lied, never stolen, never killed, never not honored me or the Creator who made her. And not once was she beaten, or yelled at or even put in "time-out." She is unconditionally loved, and knows no fear. Her connection to God is through humanity, the earth, and the universe. She judges no one. When she doesn't condone behaviors in her friends, she tries to help them learn why they behave as they do. She asks two questions before she speaks or acts. Am I coming from love, or from fear? If she is certain she is coming from love, her second question is, are my actions or words in the highest and best interest of everyone, including myself?

All actions come from either love or fear. There are no other emotions. Jealousy is the fear of not being as good as something or someone else. Anger is the result of not dealing with the fears of rejection, abandonment, or the low self-esteem, which is low self-love. Martyr energy comes from the fear of not being good enough and therefore, not appreciated.

Right back to the fear of rejection or abandonment, or of not being loved for who we are. Violence comes from unrestrained anger, which comes from the same fears.

If we can learn to ask these two questions before we do or say anything, we are closer to God and more in tune with our true spirit as loving human beings.

Once we learn these questions, we come closer to self-healing. If we fall out of balance from stress or overeating or changes we didn't think we were ready for, we can begin to find the cause. Did we overeat because we were afraid? Many would answer that they just liked the way the food tasted and couldn't stop. Think again. If the food tasted so good, were we afraid we wouldn't get enough or that we may never have that taste again or that someone else would get more and leave us none? If we're out of balance and blame it on stress, what is the real cause? Stress is a part of life. The body needs stress for the cells to function and for movement. When we feel stress, where is it really coming from? Are we afraid we're not working hard enough to keep our jobs? Are we fearful the money we make from the work we're doing, the work we don't love doing, isn't enough to buy the things that would make us happier than our work does? If we truly loved our work, would it make us feel stressed?

Go back to your earth walk. Every tree is your steeple, every sunset your stained glass window. Kneel, sit, or lie on the ground and feel Mother Earth cradle you. Cloud walk the shapes and messages in the sky, and speak to the rocks that steadfastly surround you. If a stranger comes upon your path, embrace him. If you hear gossip or lies or deceitful thoughts, close your ears to those vibrations. Listen instead to the music of the rain or the wind or the birds. If your legs or feet hurt, ask them why. Are you afraid to take the next step? Are you afraid to make the changes that will give you peace and happiness? If your back hurts, go back to the time it didn't hurt at all. What happened in your past that you are so fearful of letting go? Who, including yourself, have you not forgiven?

Why do you feel you have to carry the troubles of others? Who put you in charge of someone else's life? If your stomach aches, ask why you are having trouble digesting what you see or hear or feel. If you have allergies, ask why you are allergic to the world around you. Are you filled with the same toxic waste that now fills the earth? If your child has allergies or is considered ADHD, are you filling her with the same toxins you ingest? Have you shown her you're not afraid to love so she can also know that love is not anger or coldness or hate or frustration? Are you feeding yourself the bounty of the earth without first having it processed? We process all information, all feelings, and all sensations through our brain instead of our hearts. Unprocess your food and water so your body can know which poisons to fight.

Have faith that your spirit is a part of the Divine energy that gave you life and take the time to know that spirit. Embrace it without fear.

To know your spirit is the peace that faith gives us. Believe. With all your heart, with all your soul. The seventh key allows the power of all the others.

CONCLUSION

The life and health of your body is your strongest connection to earth, and you have a responsibility to make it present, keep it balanced, and allow it to thrive. The cause of all illness, all imbalance, is within us. Our tissues remember, our brains have filed away each step, each occurrence, and our hearts beat the song of every misguided choice. Our fingernails are ten red flags that reach out every day to send us needed messages. Our eyes have recorded every bump, scrape, and broken bone, and our chakras have dimmed with every unresolved or uncleared trauma.

We were meant to take into our bodies all that is good, and to discard the waste that God knew we would create. We were meant to drink and bathe in clean water and absorb its vibration, its essence. We were meant to touch each other with kindness, knowing that every touch that comes from a loving heart is a healing touch, not only for those who receive, but for the giver as well. We were meant to speak our words carefully as God taught with the speaking of His own words, and to listen to the vibration of the words of others with open ears and loving hearts. We were meant to know our reflection, and to know that we are a reflection of our creator, a reflection of heaven. We were meant to judge only ourselves in relation to our choices on earth, and to automatically, unconditionally, forgive the frailty of all who touch our lives. We were meant to harbor the soul and its intention, and to keep that harbor free of resentment, distrust, anger, or fear. We were meant to recreate ourselves, not in our own image, but in the image of our higher, and then highest self and to earn our wings by allowing others to earn theirs. We were meant to love. With every breath, every blink, every tear, every action, every word-not only ourselves-but to love every creature, every being, every creation in our world. We were meant to know the difference between energy that comes from fear, and that which comes from love, and to know that only through the love that emanates from us can we truly see the reflection of that love. We were meant to be well, and to walk the earth for as many years as we need to serve our original purpose.

These are the things that stop our walk:

Inoculations: Our own, and those given to our children. Though considered preventative, they are the poisons that will torment our bodies until death.

Polluted water: Drinking it, bathing in it, allowing our children to swim in it. That pollution is all man-made, and the man-made chemicals that we believe protect us are just as, if not more, dangerous. Chlorine and chlorine by-products are deadly. Bromide may be a solution for swimming pools and spas. Multi-stage purifiers are no longer luxuries.

Processed or chemical-laden food: We have been given every form of nourishment our entire being needs to not only survive, but also to flourish. We have a responsibility to learn about all the food the earth provides and to use it wisely.

Fluoride toothpaste, deodorants, and make-up: Read the ingredients and know that using these products creates a chemical factory within every tissue and cell.

Television, Radio, video games, computers: Not only do these inventions cause stagnation in our children, but also the posture of the participants causes misalignment in the neck and back, radiation poisoning, and a detachment from the earth.

The programming also causes static vibrations which interfere with many of the normal processes of the body. The content of the programs is usually negative and promotes fear or apathy.

Synthetic supplements and vitamins: These are laboratory concoctions that don't contain the natural sources of nutrition provided by the earth, and are often coated with sugar or sugar-free chemicals.

Artificial sweeteners: Joint pain, arthritis, bloating, colon problems and memory loss are the by-products of artificial sweeteners.

Synthetic clothing: The chemicals within the fabric of synthetic clothing are absorbed through our skin and exacerbated by the chemicals in the detergents we use.

Soda: Caffeinated soda attacks the heart, adrenal glands, pituitary and the liver and kidneys. The phosphorus content is so high in carbonated drinks that it would take a nine hundred pound person to properly absorb and use the contents of one eight ounce can.

Coffee and coffee substitutes: These are diuretics that not only cause fluid loss in an already dehydrated society, but also leech calcium from the tissues and bones and deposit that calcium in the kidneys.

Shoes, especially high heels, flip-flops and any shoe without arch supports: Our feet are a microcosm of our body and contain the map to every organ and system. Without proper support, our arches and heels suffer, which in turn weakens the associated parts of the body.

Antacids: If we eat eighty percent alkaline and twenty percent acid, we don't need antacids. If we do have a Ph imbalance, adding apple cider vinegar before a meal may alleviate any symptoms of indigestion.

Pain relievers: Pain is a gift. It tells us we are doing something wrong and need to change. Masking pain leads to accelerated or alternative symptoms as the body tries to communicate the problem. Find the cause of the pain instead, and then make the changes. Aches or pains that come from exercise or body work can be alleviated by adding a cup or two of apple cider vinegar to a full bathtub and soaking for twenty minutes. The bathwater, of course, should be healthy water.

Medications: Laboratory, man-made interventions that deter us from finding the cause of an illness and most of the time cause an acidic condition in the body that encourages more disease. We all need an occasional "jump start" when we're out of balance, but we are a world dependant on these crutches, rather than a humanity who learns how to be well.

Food combinations: Even if we eat only the finest, purest food, we will have digestive disorders if we combine these foods incorrectly, or overindulge in them. Improper combining causes acidic conditions and internal fermentation.

Fast Food: Fast food equals a faster death. Loaded with trans fats, wheat gluten and very acidic. Have a fast vegetable instead.

Microwave ovens: Microwaving food, coffee and water changes the molecular structure, which will also change your molecular structure.

Plastic bottles, soda cans, birth control products, medications, garbage: All of these things get buried in landfills which then leak into our water tables and get recycled into our bodies.

Fungus & Mold: Most prevalent in the southeastern United States, but rapidly spread by weather systems. Some of the best ways to fight these insidious intruders is with therapeutic grade essential oils, particularly oregano. We recommend Young Living oils as they are exceptional grade and trustworthy. Also, use Vicks on toenail fungus.

Pillows: Body alignment during sleep is extremely important in the natural healing process. We do most of our healing while at rest. We rely on fluffy pillows and crooked arms to support our heads and necks, instead of supporting the natural curvature of our spines.

Language: Our words create. Our language, the way we speak to each other, and the words we accept from others, can be a negative challenge, or a positive reinforcement.

OPIUM: Other People's Influence Under Mining your health. Pay attention to your own heart and intuition. Get educated. We are addicted to one pill answers and so-called miracle cures. What supposedly worked for your neighbor may not work for you

Automobiles: They have done a great job convincing us that we need cars to survive. No longer a luxury, cars have caused us to be lazy and careless, especially when people feel the need to eat, drink or talk on the phone while driving. We need to walk, or find ways to use our legs to accomplish our tasks. If we can't, then we need to change our work, change our schedules, change our lives.

Attitudes and Egos: No one of us is better than or more important than the other. We are snowflakes and fingerprints, each different and unique, each with a different purpose. There is no power in attitude. There is no honor in ego. The use and abuse of either of these is negative energy that attacks the giver and the receiver. Go back to the two basic questions and check the ego or the attitude.

Belief: If you believe your faith, your church, or your God is better than anyone else's, find your true spirit and change your belief. This has always been and still is one of the biggest killers in our world.

We only have one chance to do our earth walk, as continuous as it may seem, or as terrible as it seems to so many. The gift of life is the true miracle. It may come wrapped in different colors and be adorned with many different decorations. It may be challenged by what seem to be insurmountable obstacles, or by incorrigible angels placed in our path. We were meant to live, and you have all the keys. You may not be able to do everything, but you can try. You may not succeed in all you try, but you can try again. A percentage of feeling better, is better than you are right now. Embrace your life. Honor it with all your might by trying to do all that is in the highest interest of the body, mind, and spirit that allow you to be. Forget the cures. Find the cause and truly live.

Printed in the United States
68011LVS00007B/9